I REJECTED BYPASS SURGERY FOR A BETTER LIFE

BY

Robert A. Gegan

Author of "How to Attain Total Wellness"

CONSUMER INFORMATION PUBLICATIONS, INC.
P.O. Box 6203
Clearwater, Fla. 33518

cip
BOOKS

DEDICATION

To my oldest son, Bob . . . who searched and found a remarkable alternative to bypass surgery in Chelation Therapy. Through his own trials and tribulations with stomach cancer, he took time to research and advise me.

His loving & grateful Dad

To the thousands of heart patients who have undergone bypass surgery, and to the millions more with coronary vascular disease, and to the still millions more who do not know as yet that they have this progressive disease, I dedicate this vital message.

Your devoted reporter

To my cardiologist . . . who was most helpful with explainations, care and advice; but too quick and casual in recommending bypass surgery soon. Through his actions, I sought and found a better and safe way, Chelation Therapy.

His grateful patient

To the American Academy of Medical Preventics for their cooperation and help in compiling information and advice on Chelation Therapy as well as preventive medicine. To all the encouragement and advice from Dr.'s Joe Horowitz, Bob Rogers and Elmer Cranton.

With deepest thanks,

Robert A. Gegan

CONTENTS

"HE WHO HAS HEALTH HAS HOPE; AND HE THAT HAS HOPE HAS EVERYTHING."

. . . Arabian proverb.

Library of Congress #81-66843

ISBN #0-940062-01-1

First Printing 2/81
Second Printing 11/81

FOREWORD

"Thanks - your book saved my life!" Those are the greatest words I hear from the public, and I hear them regularly when I travel. I also receive hundreds of letters explaining how nutrition and chelation therapy have made well persons out of inoperable sickly patients.

Bob Gegan was one such individual whom I had the pleasure to meet at a conference in Ft. Lauderdale, Florida. I was pleased not only because he was well and vibrant, but because by writing this book he was going to tell others how they might be helped. Bob Gegan has done an excellent job of bringing new information on chelation therapy and nutrition to you. He clearly explains what worked for him to gain freedom from heart disease. Perhaps some day you will walk up to him and say, "Thanks, your book saved my (or a friend's) life."

Only a physician who has examined you can give a qualified judgement regarding your best treatment. However, many physicians have not studied chelation therapy or nutrition and they don't trust what they don't understand. Most physicians who do study chelation therapy and nutrition go on to use them as their first choices in treatment.

If you have heart disease, you owe it to your family and to yourself to be examined by a physician who is a qualified chelation therapist. This book will help you understand the alternatives. You are responsible for your health, so choose advisers who offer you the best options.

Richard Passwater, Ph.D.
Author-Nutritionist-Researcher
Berlin, MD

FOREWORD II

There definitely is a safe and effective alternative to bypass surgery, despite what you may have learned from other sources!

Nevertheless, cardiologists and cardiovascular surgeons continue to aggressively endorse the treatment of occlusive coronary artery disease and of other vascular blockages with highly invasive and very expensive by-pass surgery. Surgical treatment involves considerable risk of death and of other complications, and is usually recommended to patients without the slightest mention of the alternative, intravenous disodium ethylene diamine tetraacetic acid (EDTA) chelation therapy. Chelation therapy is far less expensive, far safer and is most frequently just as effective as surgery, in relieving symptoms of diminished blood flow.

Arteriograms followed by by-pass surgery comprise a major medical industry in the United States.

Medical centers are coming to rely on these high sources of income to subsidize their operations. Hospitals are becoming dependent on income from by-pass surgery and related procedures literally, for their survival.

If chelation therapy is truly as safe and as effective as indicated by recent scientific studies, many catheter-trained cardiologists and an increasting number of cardiovascular surgeons must drastically mofidy their methods of treatment. Perhaps these facts explain why chelation therapy has been so slow to gain acceptance and why there persists a closed-minded attitude in opposition to chelation therapy by certain segments of the medical profession.

I have personally been using EDTA chelation therapy in my practice for more than seven years. I have observed hundreds of patients benefit greatly from this treatment. Angina and other heart problems have improved. Legs have been saved from amputation and senility has been reversed. My success rate with this therapy exceeds 75 percent, and approaches 90 percent in those patients who correct their dietary, exercise and smoking habits which are known to aggravate occlusive vascular disease. Symptoms improve, blood flow to diseased organs increases and, most importantly, the quality of life is greatly enhanced. Many such patients have exhausted all other available treatments before coming for chelation therapy. I have not seen any serious complications or side effects when chelation therapy is properly administered by a physician who is expert in its use. Patients have frequently come to me after the failure of one or more by-pass surgeries, and even in those cases chelation therapy has often been effective. Tens of thousands of patients who have been successfully treated with chelation therapy have now become enthusiastic advocates. Robert A. Gegan, the author of this book, is one such former patient who writes from personal experience.

Segments of the medical profession, governmental bureaucracies and the medical insurance industry have consistently attempted to suppress and persecute this therapy. They have blocked reimbursement for chelation therapy by Medicare, by other federally-funded insurance programs and by most private insurance companies. Physicians have been threatened with loss of their licenses to practice merely for using chelation therapy. Hospital staffs routinely refuse to allow this treatment on hospitalized patients.

The same medical insurance companies which refuse to pay for chelation therapy, pay without question for the much more expensive by-pass surgeries. Physician consultants to medical insurance companies seem to have a vested interest in maintaining the status quo. Newer and far less expensive therapies, such as chelation, have been unjustly discriminated against.

Is it possible that chelation therapy has been suppressed in an attempt to maintain a monopoly by vascular surgeons on the treatment of diminished blood flow? Any such attempt to unfairly restrain the practice of physicians using chelation therapy would be in distinct violation of restraint of trade laws and would certainly be in opposition to the best interests of the American public.

Those physicians who have openly criticized the safety and effectiveness of chelation therapy have done so without benefit of personal experience using this therapy. They rely entirely on obsolete scientific studies and professional bias in their attacks on chelation therapy. They have, on occasion, misrepresented published research to support their stance in opposition to chelation therapy.

Two scientific studies by H. Richard Casdorph, M.D., Ph.D., Assistant Clinical Professor of Medicine at the University of California, Irvine, California, have been recently accepted for publication in the **Journal of Holistic Medicine.** One study concerns the successful use of EDTA chelation therapy in coronary artery disease and the other describes dramatic improvement in brain disease and senility. Both studies were subjected to strict statistical analysis and the results proved to be highly significant, with a probability that the same results could have occurred by mere chance of less than 5 in 10,000 (P0 .005). These studies were scientifically controlled by doing before and after measurements of blood flow in every patient—the patients themselves acted as their own controls.

The American Academy of Medical Preventics, an organization of holistic physicians, sets professional standards for the use of EDTA chelation therapy. The American Holistic Medical Association has sponsored workshops and speakers on this new and important form of therapy. One such recent speaker is John H. Olwin, M.D., Clinical Professor of Surgery Emeritus at Rush Medical College, University of Illinois, and attending vascular surgeon at St. Luke's Presbyterian Hospital in Chicago, who has for many years utilized intravenous EDTA chelation therapy with great success on patients with blocked arteries. It is estimated that more than a thousand physicians across the country have been using this therapy with a high degree of safety and effectiveness for more than two decades. Nevertheless, EDTA chelation therapy is still suppressed and has been prevented from widespread acceptance by critics who claim that it is "quackery" and "dangerous"—falsely implying that by-pass surgery is comparatively safer and more effective.

Bob Gegan has performed a great public service in this book by relating his own personal experiences with chelation therapy. He has thoroughly researched and reported the facts concerning chelation and he also describes many other ways to slow or to reverse the adverse effects of aging. Highly beneficial and cost effective techniques of improved nutrition, physical exercise conditioning, metabolic therapies and stress management are all described in a way which will stimulate the discerning reader to make life-style changes to prevent the need for crisis intervention after a heart attack, stroke or other health catastrophy has occurred.

I highly recommend this book. What worked for Bob Gegan can work for you

Elmer M. Cranton, M.D.
Trout Dale, Virginia
President,
American Holistic Medical Association

INTRODUCTION

I am going to let you in on a little known secret . . . your possible interest in a growing $80 billion industry. This is no get-rich-quick scheme and it appears the income will rise sharply for many more years. If you want in, it's easy. All you need to do is stop reading this book right now, and you are on your way into the largest boon-doggle in medical history . . . the business of bypass surgery. It is now a four billion dollar business and predicted to grow by 1986 to 80 billion dollars yearly. So if you put this book back on the shelf and go about your life as usual, your prospects are good for joining this big industry . . . as a contributor.

I gave a copy of the original edition of this book to some friends. They reported to me that some friends of theirs upon visiting their home, spotted my book. My good friends had not read the book themselves as yet, but their friends both had occlusive heart disease and the husband had undergone bypass surgery. The book title "rang the bell" and these nice people practically insisted on borrowing the book as they "just needed to read it."

They were very prompt in returning the book and were asked how they liked it. Their answer gave my good friends (and later me) a jolt. "We asked our doctor about chelation therapy and he said to forget it, it is a non-approved therapy that has been around for years, so we did not bother to read it."

And so, dear reader, if you are going to be foolish enough to believe what your doctor tells you about the contents of this book . . . all true facts, I assure you . . . then you have been taken in also by untrue stories. So there's no use purchasing this book, even though it can save your life. Better still, give the purchase price to your church . . you may need the prayerful benefits the Lord may bestow on you.

On the other hand, the facts related in the following pages give me pleasure beyond description . . . as I am able to help people discover that there is a better way to a healthy and enjoyable life. I am talking about people who have been told there's nothing more that can be done for them, people who have been "put out to pasture" for their remaining years, people who sit home disabled from heart disease. I have talked to many of them and, believe it or not, some want to be helped and others just don't think it's possible. What a pity.

Many people so afflicted will read this book but do nothing to help themselves. They seem resigned to their eventual fate or are just not convinced enough to take their destiny into their own hands. I am told by doctors that there are millions like that. "You can lead a horse to water, but you can't make him drink," really holds true of some people. Desire . . . can make life enjoyable again. It is my aim to instill this desire in you if you will give me the chance.

You see, I was a victim of my own bad habits and lifestyle. The doctors just love anyone who dissipates like I did. Their business booms from hopeless victims like myself, and people who are victims of their own bad habits.

You see, I am just a typical old traveling salesman who was scared out of his skin by a sudden heart attack. My experiences will prove beneficial to everyone who reads this book. This is my contribution, my legacy to mankind, my thanks for joyful living again.

Many of you have read the book or remember the movie, "Death of a Salesman". The principal character resembles me and my life over the past thirty years. I am told the scenario for the book was written around Lima, Ohio, life. That, too, was an old stomping ground of mine as I traveled around that state for 20 years.

No matter what night of the week any salesman would land in Lima there was always "action" there at the bars. Business was always good as word spread among all traveling men, that Lima was the place for "action" and "pickings" were easy and plentiful.

Tobacco and alcohol were my off-business constant diet. Dissipation interfered somewhat with the business routine, but foolishly, weakness and temptation allowed it to be continue. When you are master of your own destiny (no boss to account to) you take advantage of your own weaknesses. I told myself that I had to smoke to keep awake so that I would not have another near-miss accident. And smoke I did. I inhaled cigars like they were cigarettes, many more than 20 per day.

It became a real "drag" when I arrived home from towns like Lima. I had to try and get some rest, and at the same time pretend that I felt no effects from my week away in dissipation. I blamed the grueling driving and traveling conditions as my problem.

Aside from the business routine, my wife and I lived a slightly similiar lifestyle. We were members of a country club. There was golf, parties, entertaining, and the club was a "bottle Club". This means that you have a numbered bottle of whisky and you drink without ever bothering to measure what goes into the glass with your ice and water. I am sure you know the results . . . an early night into drunkeness.

In retrospect I assure you that such a week-by-week traveling diet was unhealthy, but I kept active, exercised when at home and just kept going. But in-between the greasy restaurant meals, smoking, later hours and inactive long driving, I spent some time home where a good home-cooked meal was really appreciated.

I could not stand the cold winters in Ohio. My feet and hands were always cold, and my always cold feeling created the need for warmth. So we moved to Florida.

It wasn't too long that I was on the road again, older, a little wiser (I was slowing down) but not smart enough. I inherited high blood pressure and needed to seek medical help. Since this is a doctors paradise (they are all busy) I had to seek out a new doctor who had just gone into his first practice. I took pills galore, but they did not seem to eliminate my symptoms completely. One drug was designed to keep the circulation to the brain opened, one was a diuretic, another Valium and a fourth for my constant headaches. Later for my problem of dizziness and headache the doctor prescribed Ismelin. This is where I believe all my problems started. Or was it just too many drugs?

It wasn't too long after starting Ismelin that upon waking in the night to go to the john, I keeled over on the bathroom floor. After repeated episodes of fainting or passing out I began to be concerned and came home. I then went to the doctor's office and explained my new problem to him. He changed the prescription, remarking that maybe the Ismelin was too strong. Since he was unconcerned, I asked if I should have another physical examination. The tests were started that same day and I also decided myself that I should have a treadmill test as I was worried about my condition.

The next day, a Friday, I went to the hospital for a treadmill test. I was on and off the treadmill rather quickly as I could not endure the pain in my feet and legs, any longer. The attending cardiologist remarked that he did not believe the test would reveal anything in so short a time, and I left the hospital.

The following Monday my heart attack accured. Actually, I never had a serious illness in my life. I knew nothing about diet, nutrition, hardening of the arteries or poor circulation and its causes. I gave no thought to why I had high blood pressure. I though it was a natural condition for my age. The pills were keeping the blood pressure within limits, so why worry? But I did stop smoking finally.

Over the years in my business I met many people who talked endlessly about their health problems and their operations. No matter how serious the problem of their health, I could not help being concerned and sympathetic to their problems. But unless one is very close to that person, the story is soon forgotten as passing conversation. It happens to everyone.

Now it has happened to me and I have something to talk about too. The attending cardiologist in the cardiac care unit at the hospital said the heart attack could be the best thing that every happened to me . . . I had a warning . . . to "straighten up and fly right". It was right there that my life changed. I figured at 67 years of age I could enjoy life for many more years if I had the determination to change.

PREFACE

The search for treatment by chelation therapy after my heart attack consisted of finding success stories, technical knowledge and a physician to administer it here in Florida. Information was sparce, but after a while things gradually came into focus.

The second part was the investigation of why the American Medical Association (AMA) did not endorse the treatment, and more importantly why the Federal Government would not pay for the treatments under Medicare. All this did not make good sense to me. Here was a therapy that should cost no more than a tenth of the cost of bypass surgery. It cleans out all the arteries from the top of your head to the tip of your toes. It is not just a serious relief operation that leaves ugly scars on your chest and may have to be performed again sometime later. I was puzzled, because if you balance the benefits of chelation against bypass surgery, there's no contest; chelation wins by a wide margin . . . so, back to my reading binge.

I was fortunate to be sent various articles from friends and relatives. They were for and against bypass surgery that I was told was needed if I wish to live a normal life again. I was not impressed with the results I read about, since all that I could really find out for sure was it relieved angina pain.

The first book I read on the subject was *Supernutrition, The Megavitamin Revolution,* by Richard Passwater, PhD. The cover of the book states: You can have the kind of energy and vibrant health you never dreamed possible. The list of renoned doctors in the acknowedgements were staggering.

It was then suggested that I then read Passwater's latest book, *Supernutrition For Health Hearts.* Its front cover states: "Your heat can be five years younger in three months, ten years younger in nine months, with this revolutionary six-step program." Passwater has a wealth of research to back up all the facts and in particular the most important truth of all . . . dietary cholesterol does *not* cause heart disease. (There goes my egg beaters diet). In fact, Passwater declares that "if anyone can step forward to prove that eating cholesterol does cause heart disease, I will donate all the proceeds of this book to the American Heart Association."

I strongly recommend both of Passwater's books for their completeness and research in the cholesterol conflict, nutrition and vitamin E.

Conventional medicine must assume most of the blame for its lack of knowledge about nutrition and vitamins. Many times members of the profession will react negatively to the subject . . . while the truth may be that they know little about it. This may result from mis-information passed on through the AMA Journal and a deficiency in training in the medical schools until recent years.

As a result, many times a doctor reacts with "protectionism", that is, only he (or government) has your personal interest in mind; have faith in him, you cannot go wrong listening to his advice. This he theorizes, and often defends with the catch-word, "quackery", in his statements. Who **are** these men in the white coats?

The story is almost the same with chelation therapy. The AMA knows little about it (they say) but they must assume the same blame for ignorance as with nutrition rather than the individual non-member doctors.

This book has among its objectives the following:

- the prevention of heart attack
- the alternative to bypass surgery
- an aid to stroke victims
- the serious problems of stress
- a solution to senility and mental problems
- an aid to arthritis victims
- the problems of our water
- a cure for gangrene induced by diabetes
- living proof of chelation therapy's success
- our total health and happiness
- details of discoveries that may help readers
- the unfounded adamant AMA opposition
- predictability and prevention of all serious diseases
- National Health Reformation

This book is also a layman-to-layman narration, trying to eliminate fancy terms; many doctors use them by talking over your head. I may occassionally slip into technical wording, but that's explained in the glossary in the back of the book.

I have researched many books, reports, reprints, studies, etc., all written by experts in their fields. They are physicians, research scientists and nutritionists renowned in their fields. Sometimes we hear stories that recommend but do not tell why. I want to know all the W's, the whos, the whens, the wheres and the whys so I can make my own judgment on the merits of any recommendation. I wish to ease the reader's mind with simple information, in order to help heal his or her bodies.

I must warn you though (as I found out) you will have to change your lifestyle. You will discover that nature heals, not the physician . . . and that it is possible to help heal yourself. I assure you, it will be well worth the eventual rewards.

Reading constantly, I have learned the laws of the human body and how to apply them. This is one qualification I have for these written contents. The second qualification for this written word is my own vitality and endurance at sixty-eight years of age, after a serious heart attack. Of course, I learned later how to reverse this debilitative disease. This was a major project for me, and the important knowledge for everyone to have and cherish.

As I constantly endure this writing task and delve deeply into all the various subjects, I know that this effort will be worthwhile if just one reader's life will be spared or just one reader will be motivated to exert the extra effort to modify his/her current lifestyle and to acquire and maintain a healthy and happy existence.

Chapter One

PLEASE MR. PRESIDENT

The gift of happiness belongs to those who "unwrap" it.
. . . Andrew Dunbar.

The President of the United States
The White House
1600 Pennsylvania Ave.
Washington, D.C.

Dear Mr. President:

If ever there was a time when every one of us would begin to realize that we must participate in our own search for health care, it is now. We are shackled into spending on "designed" health care well over 200 billion dollars yearly. To make matters worse, with the present design, such staggering costs are doing little good as we seem to go backwards and continue to pay more and more each year for less and less in real effective health care. We cannot blame it all on inflation either, as we are in a financial crisis in health care maintanence.

In 1980 pollster Louis Harris found that 62 percent of the population felt their lives were **out of control.** Only one in five Americans have faith in their representation of government, medicine, religion or business.

I am sounding off, Mr. President, as I have personally learned the hard way, (as you read my book) that I am alarmed. Alarmed that my own personal illness could have ended tragically and possibly purposely; that millions of Americans like myself are being discriminated against both financially and medically by government; that heart disease problems alone are costing government 80 billion dollars every year needlessly; and worst of all, most afflicted people with various other diseases, continue to suffer and pay needlessly. As we now find out, preventive measures were the real answer.

During my extensive reading I became convinced we are victims of design and conspiracy. The enemy is conventional or organized medicine represented by The American Medical Association (AMA) who in turn strongly influence government into protectionism tactics that accomplish little or nothing but higher medical bills. They talk a "good game" but results are lacking. The overly restrictive guidelines of the FDA is an example.

For generations this august body has insisted in trying to control our lives. They persist in treating symptoms, as Americans become used to leaning on drugs, rather than achieving a cure (this is the design I speak about). They attempt to "play father" to us when we really don't need them. Their treatment of diseases is seldom permanent or effective and the number of drugs prescribed are often more dangerous than the illness they are designed to treat. They have grown to a designed creed of "have faith in me, doctor knows best." Our health care values keep diminishing and conventional medicine is slowly losing dominance over the American people who are slowly learning prevention.

It is not fair to those people practicing prevention. Why should we reward illness and penalize wellness? Particularly since we have answers to most preventive measures that we practice. Isn't it better Mr. President to think about economic incentives for people to stay healthy?

Here are just four brief description areas of medical treatment where conventional medicine really has no effective treatment, but where there are some answers:

DISEASE	**CONVENTIONAL SOLUTIONS**	**PREVENTIVE MEDICINE SOLUTIONS**
Gangrene	Usually Amutation of limb	Restore circulation with chelation therapy and possibly hyperbaric oxygen therapy, diet, exercise and nutrition.
Schizophrenia, Memory Loss & Related Problems	Psychiatry & drugs. Shock treatment, institutionalizing, tranquilizers, etc.	Same as above.
Senility, Memory Loss & Related Problems	Desecrating, depressive and submissive drugs.	Reversing the aging process as above.
Occlusive Heart Disease & Related Problems	$20,000 bypass surgery, dialating drugs, disability.	Same as above and restoring normal living. Overall improved health and noninvasive testing.

Mr. President if you have someone figure out the costs of these four diseases (and there are more) you must agree that conventional medicine and the FDA guidelines are costing us all hundreds of billions of dollars and the suffering goes on.

This is the answer to many of your budget reducing problems and we have the answers suggested in I REJECTED BYPASS SURGERY FOR A BETTER LIFE.

I note this DAN DORFMAN column headline: HOSPITAL CARE COSTS EXPECTED TO MULTIPLY: NOBODY CARES, SAY INDUSTRY CONSULTANT. Growing at an annual rate of 15 to 16 percent the fastest growing segment of the population, that of old age infirmities, make up the bulk of this problem. Predictions for future costs could make you sick just thinkg-ing about $700 per day for a semi-private room in just five years, then double again in five more years to $1400 per day.

The article in the St. Petersburg Times 6/21/81 in an interview with David M. Edwards, hospital consultant, states, "nobody gives a damn, not even Uncle Sam, who does not even bother to monitor such costs and increases."

I am worried Mr. President, about that statement and the fact that is now costs $2450 for an average 7-day stay in a hospital, and that government pays $88 Billion per year which I hope to prove in part is needless.

Of course, this is typical of inflation attitudes in general as the same percentages of profit make still higher profit from rampant increases. I wonder just who really cares. Most hospitals care less about holding down costs. The 3rd party payments of 80 percent are guaranteed, making a built-in safeguard. They have profits in abundance for new added wings, alterations, new equipment and public relations expenses.

We still are confronted with "big brother" movement of government which continues to develop new bureaucracies to write, oversee and enforce new laws that are designed to protect us from the evils that surround us. Of course as you are now finding out, the benefits are not worth the high costs, and they are almost impossible to change.

I called this rising era of indignation "protectionism." These high ideals have not worked successfully in many cases, they have affected our way of living to a point that most protectionism is harmful, getting more expensive and growing oppressive. Isn't it time every American started thinking for himself? For instance, an important action I suggest you initiate . . ., We have a dire need for freedom of choice in medicine. Why not, we are paying for it.

Bruce Stokes, a researcher for World Watch Institute, a private non-profit foundation says, "powerless people make poor citizens in a democracy." There are signs that Americans, spurred by economic pressures, are beginning to take an active interest in their own problem-solving and organizing self-help groups. Stokes says, "in the name of convenience, dependency has been turned on its head and celebrated as a virtue. People mistakeingly think that one of the benefits of affluence is that they no longer need involve themselves in such mundane activities as home repair or self-care of simple illnesses."

"It will not be easy to overcome the pervasive alienation now afflicting our society. But what better way to begin than involving people in self-help activities? And, sums up Stokes, To give people that all important sense of control over their lives."

With flying colors we went through the successful antivirus era that medical science virtually conquered. We are now nearing the end of another time frame, and degenerative disease (with design) has gained very little toward the cure of heart disease or cancer. And already the new nutritional era is upon us. This nutritional era will soon cut into the statistical stigma on our records. It is predicted that this era will put America on the road to health through biological and metabolic corrections to illness and disease. But we need your help.

Over the past decades we have spent trillions of dollars contributing to the war on cancer and heart disease . . . but to no avail. I believe by design, these diseases are still with us. Here is a futile assault on symptoms, and for thirty years there are only little "teasing" answers forthcoming. But charitable organizations do have excellent public relations ballyhoo of promises, flowered with glowing expectations that occur year after year before the start of their drives for funds. Our government spends billions, Mr. President, on support of these national organizations. Then we add more of our own dollars by public donations to support this seemingly useless waste. National Health Reformation described in later chapters can cure this problem easily, and it will not cost government anything to do.

As you will read later in my book, the government is not helping us as we seek relief from protectionism. Again we and government are being influenced by the "gods in the white coats" and such shackles must be broken before our health care costs sends us into bancrupcy.

What can we do? We need to seek out and find the new unselfish doctors who share our regard for life, and who use their skills to protect and extend our lives happily. We can't choose when we die, but we should choose how long we live.

Its time such worthy groups were recognized as prominent meaningful medical societies, Mr. President. I call them splinter groups from the AMA. These groups of physicians will help cut billions of dollars of our health maintanence costs. Their attention to health is decidely different and highly effective. I know. They practice prevention, use less drugs, use the holistic approach to treating the entire body and know nutrition as a metabolic cure. They are gaining strength fast and I predict they will eventually outnumber the membership of the AMA who have selfishly opposed them for many years.

As they break away from AMA old fashioned belief, these same groups of professionals dare to oppose the AMA; they dare to cure; they dare to suffer from radical harrassment and oppression for the sake of their beliefs and "feelings" they have for their patient's welfare. These are the groups to which the terminally afflicated go for help as a last resort. And importantly, these groups can help all sick people; they can effectively help you and Congress cut our staggering medical costs.

Since all of the above are true facts, it stands to reason we need solutions. For instance arteriosclerosis is almost completely preventable and is 95 percent reversible. This means our country's #1 killer is both preventable and reversible. We can slowly nibble away at these costs and we can reverse the basic causes. The solution lies in a National Prevention program, but the opposition has been knocking down such ideas each time they are discussed. Now wise Americans are joining hands with their new breed of medical doctor and getting answers. I believe you will not have to tangle with the congress on this program; they will get the message from their constituants. But all of you will need extreme courage and fortitude to fight the pressure of the powerful lobbies that will oppose such prevention action. I am sure the American people will be watching very closely.

Please, Mr. President. There are many more facts forthcoming as you read my book, and I know you are concerned. While you are only two years older than me, you will find out that a second term at age 74 is not insurmountable. (with some chelation therapy treatments for prevention, that would be easier) I have found now that age is just a number, its your outlook on life that affects your health. This is the area, Mr. President, of concern to millions of Americans who count on you for living out their lives with the proper happy and healthy outiook. We need you help.

Sincerely yours,

Robert A. Gegan
Author-publisher

P.S. The book, I rejected Bypass Surgery for a Better Life is being sent to you under separate cover. I hope you enjoy it. Possibly its message will be instrumental in providing budget cutting ideas.

Here are some medical groups that will help turn the tide in medical costs, There may be more:

- The American Academy of Medical Preventics
- The American Holistic Medical Association
- Academy of Orthomolecular Phychiatry
- The Northwest Academy of Preventive Medicine
- The Huxley Institute of Biosocial Research
- The Linus Pauling Institute of Science and Medicine
- The International Academy of Preventive Medicine
- International College of Applied Nutrition
- The Orthomolecular Medical Society

These groups believe that disease is in most cases a chemical imbalance, ingrained or induced, and that nutrition is chemistry. Therefore the physician should first try to correct the problem nutritionally in this science.

Dr. Robert Mendelshon, M.D., remarks in his book, *Confessions of a Medical Heretic,* when he says the patient who has no medical option to turn to (other doctor's) and submits to conventional medicine, they become frustrated and depressed. Once they find the alternative in this new medicine, they no longer regard the other side with fear and hatred. Those feelings are sometimes turned to amusement.

In order to know what these groups of physicians can do for you it is necessary to assume some responsibility for your own health care. The way your biological make-up is changed is important to you. Accordingly, I have outlined some basic facts that follow in Appendix 1.

Your request for names of the Medical Society and addresses or members near you may be had by requesting details with a stamped self envelope to: CIP Books, P.O. Box 6203, Clearwater, FL 33518.

SUMMARY THOUGHT!

The motives used in reporting my personal heart experiences, the nature of reader solutions, presents to readers a guide that is unusual in the overall theme compared to the average book. The extraneous supportive material included in the book indicates difficulties they may encounter in their quest for better health. The president's letter pinpoints overall problems as does other data, all of which were designed to try and make readers aware of and better able to cope with the problems of health care maintenance.

Chapter Two
"MY HAPPENING"

"Only the young die good".
. . . Oliver Herford

It was the following Monday morning after the Friday treadmill tests and while making my first sales call, I began to have indigestion pains.

It was during this stressful and fruitless call that I began to silently ponder the problems of pain . . . but I soon realized that I had no breakfast, so why indigestion pains? The lady prospect had no indigestion pills so I settled for a glass of water. I sat quietly awhile and finally told the lady that I felt something was wrong with me. The pain was lasting much too long and there were other little things starting to happen inside me. I told her that I may be having a heart attack and asked her if she would drive my car past the hospital on the way to my office. Then on the way I can decide how I feel and make a judgment at that time.

My new chauffeur proceeded to drive through traffic and I suddenly began to get more pain in the chest and it worked up my arm and into my back. As I broke out in a sweat and my breathing quickened, I told her to step on it right to the hospital. Unfortunately, the lady became concerned and excited as she narrowly missed some cars in some fast passing episodes. By this time my breathing came in short rapid and gasping movements and it was difficult to catch my breath.

We arrived at the hospital miraculously without incident as I told her to call my office. I walked into the emergency room and told the nurse I was having a heart attack and she asked me how I knew I was having one. Then it became obvious and she had me on a table in no time at all. People were working over me taking tests, removing clothing, ask-

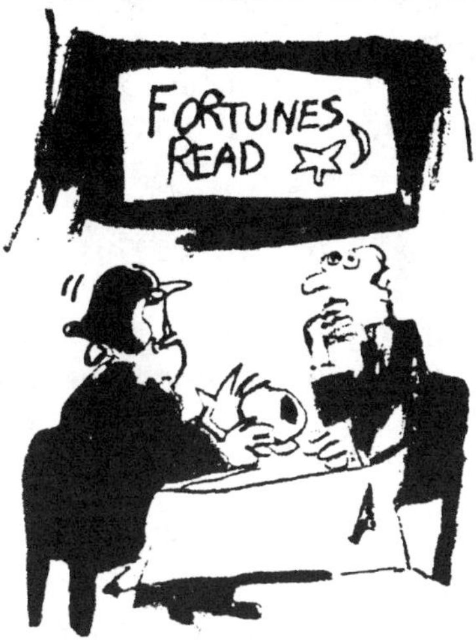

"An attractive girl will shortly take an interest in you, . . . she's a nurse in the intensive care ward."

ing questions, having me sign papers, finding a doctor to admit me and so many frantic things that had everyone around me very concerned. In about 20 minutes I was lying in bed in the cardiac care unit literally scared to death.

Some time later I was feeling much safer with all the attention I was getting from doctors and nurses as I was "wired for sound". About an hour later I was feeling relieved as I calmed down and was able to watch the monitor . . . I was confident I was in good hands.

Thirteen days later I was home and a very busy man. I was not used to the clock-work reconditioning regimen as my good wife took over completely. There was the leisurely walk with my wife twice a day, pills to take (it seemed) continuously, nitroglycerine patches to apply every few hours, food to try in a new diet and then time . . . time for reading, plenty of it. I had some catching up to do. I needed to find out about my heart condition, what caused the pain and what lay ahead for the rest of my life.

I found out that constant attention to one's health is wrought with problems and time consuming. It is also frustrating when you are not used to "must" situations. All the various schedules are orchestrated with something like food, drugs, vitamins, and new habits that sometimes taxes my dear wife's endurance. Of course, the whole idea is to relieve the angina pain, start down a new road in life while gaining back strength.

For those of you who know little about the problem (it's the #1 killer) it is caused by the lack of oxygen being delivered to the heart muscle. The medicine dialates the blood vessels and the pain usually disappears when the oxygen supply in the blood is improved. This is also helped by rest.

The entire circulatory system consists of the heart and two systems of arteries and veins interconnected by capillary networks. The arteries supply the whole body with oxygenated blood. The veins take the used blood to the lungs to be oxygenated again. This is a closed system or recirculating system using the blood over and over again. In between it is being cleansed in some areas and saturated with nutrients in other areas so that it can carry on its functions of feeding and removing waste products from the tissues and cells. The problem of feeding nutrients and removing waste is the basic cause of most all our illnesses.

The arteries carry used blood to the lungs to be oxygenated, and the veins carry oxygenated blood back to the heart to be sent into circulation to provide oxygen to the tissues and cells. The heart pumps about 4,300 gallons of blood through the body per day. This is about 100,000 heart contractions in a day's time, at a pulse rate of approximately 70 per minute.

This life sustaining process is also necessary to continue the proliferation of living cells in the body, the "key" is oxygen needed to sustain life in any form we know. We can live without food for 40 days, without water for fewer days however oxygen deprivation causes irreversible brain damage after about four minutes.

When the pumping or circulating mechanism becomes defective or the flow lines become restricted, we are in serious trouble. We have to decide to treat or cure the problem with the best medical means and advice we are able to find. This is the area where conventional medicine and the new breed of modern physicians differ on the therapy to provide us.

The arteries are arranged by Mother Nature with incredible cleverness into a complicated branching system of remarkably efficient blood-transporting tissues.

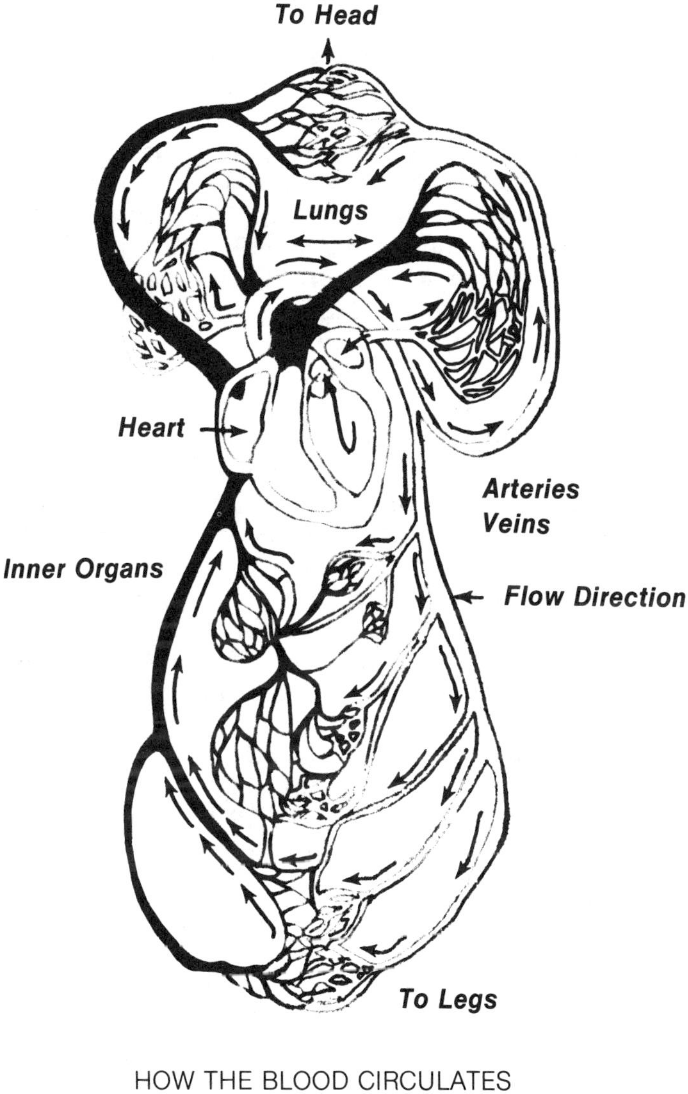

HOW THE BLOOD CIRCULATES

Showing the course of the blood through the arteries, from the heart to the rest of the body; through the veins from the tissues of the body back to the heart.

Arteries participate actively in every body function, and their functioning is of great significance to the body's well being. Arteries react to cold, heat, emotion, altitude, nervous strain, food and gravity. They are not fixed like plastic tubes; they "give" and are flexible.

The farther the blood flow from the heart, the smaller the artery channel becomes and the flow rate decreases as the vessle walls become thinner. Tiny vessels or capillaries are 50 times thinner than a human hair. The tiny corpuscles have to pass single file through the capillary. About 700 capillaries can be packed into an area the size of a shaft of a pin. If all the capillaries of the body were placed end to end they would form a thread-like tube passing several times around the earth.

About one-quarter of the blood moving in the body is found in the lungs. The surface of all the lung cells is about 1200 square yards which is constantly exposed to air in the lungs. The surface of the lungs is not stationary. Like a giant cylinder of living tissue, fresh air moves past the chambers of the lungs and is absorbed in the blood, more like a spongy wheel picks up water. Every second, two billion blood cells pass the air chambers of the lungs; so this living tissue captures and binds atmospheric air, part of which is pure oxygen.

As blood flows, it is renewed as are the cells of the body. Even as you read this page, parts of yesterday's physical body is to change and vanish. Your body parts today are both appearing and disappearing; tomorrow's bones, muscles and glands are still being created. Much of the body's physical health is up to you and how you care for it. Your blood chemistry is influenced by your eating habits. Hence the need to emphasize the "quality" of what we eat.

It was about two months later that I was able to go to a new doctor, a cardiologist. Here I learned a little about the attack and how the heart works, I found out that I soon would be ready for some tests to see how good (or bad) the problem was to become.

The doctor planned before the next visit that I should be in good enough shape from the prescribed exercise, rest and drug therapy for a stress cardigram. Well at the witching hour, I had the tests and I was on and off the treadmill in no time at all, it seemed, and I flunked the test miserably. The doctor remarked that possibly the tests were premature, even though he determined the time lag. But he did not schedule another treadmill test later.

Still later on in time I agreed to take a catheteration or cath test. I found out after the tests that this is a dangerous procedure involving inserting a plastic tube through the blood vessel right up to the heart and injecting dye right into the arteries entering the heart, while at the same time taking pictures of the traveling dye entering the heart. Luckily all went well.

Before leaving the hospital I received the bad news . . . three blockages. The cardiologist immediately recommended bypass surgery as if it were nothing more than repairing a broken arm. "And while it is a serious operation, it is being done every day", and I should condensend if I wanted to live a normal life again.

As suggested by the cardiologist my wife and I went to see one of the surgeons on the team and after his review of the cath pictures he said it looked like four blockages. He explained the operation in a matter-of-fact way with brief details most casually. I found out that Medicare paid for the "majority" of the bill and that the costs amounted to about the price of a sports car. He did not say what sports car but I am sure he meant an expensive foreign one. I was not particularly pleased with the interruptions and the short conversations, and I had a quick reply to the question the surgeon put to me. "Shall I set up a hospital date for you?" Just as though an immediate decision was a common practice, my answer was yes and no. No you cannot set up a date and yes I want to think this all over. And *think I did.*

At that time I was doubly disappointed and disgusted with my condition as well as the two specialists recommendation. I have not been back to see either man again.

PRECAUTIONARY MEASURES

One of the first things I read about was the rate of recurrence of another heart attack. The 45 percent rate worried me a little. But speaking of worry, that is very stressful, and I would rather know the higher odds against me and take meaningful steps to reduce them as low as possible. I would not want that worry on my mind constantly.

You should start asking questions during the first contacts with your doctor and before you need to make any decisions, particularly if surgery is suggested. Find out what the operation is supposed to accomplish and how it is performed. Are there any alternatives to surgery? And of course, what will happen if you do not have surgery. Then there is the chance you are taking that the operation will succeed or not, and the odds on past performance of that particular surgeon. How will the operation help or not help you, depending on your decision. With all these alternatives there are bound to be conflicts of opinion, so dig deeply.

The one basic way for awareness to work for you is to seek a second opinion by another cardiologist some time after your heart attack. Second opinions, and sometimes a third, are being paid for by insurance carriers and government. Often county medical societies will offer referral advice. The Health and Human Services maintains a toll free number (1-800-325-6400) to assist individuals in locating a specialist near his home. They recognize the element of risk from opinions and deem it cheaper in the long run. However, be careful that the second opinion may end up a rubber stamp of the first, and that you are fully informed about risks of any therapy or procedure.

Do not ask for second opinions from any doctor connected in any way with your present doctor by practice or hospital affiliation; go out of town if you must. But even then you need to ask questions and demand answers.

If the opinions differ you should go back to the first doctor and have him explain his opposing view of the second doctor or vice versa. By narrowing down the differences in opinion you will surely feel more comfortable with your own decision. But let's hope that this book can influence you also.

Tell your doctor you wish to be very frank with him and he with you. Tell him he is free to diagnose even if it gives you cause for alarm. Such opinions can be most assuring to your mental state, no matter the results. At the very least you can end up with two opinions much alike; that would also relieve even more stress. Proper mental attitude should help you change for the better.

Surgery rates in the United States have outraced the rate of population growth by three to one . . . 20,754,000 operations says the National Center of Health Statistics. A more controversial trend is the number of surgeons, a 19 percent increase in eight years, up to 1978. Dr. James Richards, an Orlando, Florida surgeon, says, The larger number of surgeons indicate more borderline operations will be done. So second opinions are important.

Contingency planning should be considered. Train yourself to avoid situations that could trigger another heart attack. Learn physiological ways to practice getting around routine and bad habits. We all have them.

Rehearsal for emergencies. This should be part of the new routine for survival. Suppose you only had 10 to 15 minutes to live from another heart attack. Know what you and your family are going to do in this emergency: oxygen, nitro pills, doctor's emergency phone number, who in the family has learned CPR (cardio pulmonary resusitation). This should be a must in every household since it is so easy to learn and definitely saves lives. Then there is the local emergency medical or paramedic team that is equipped for most any type of emergency. Mark down all the phone numbers and keep near the telephone, displayed prominently.

Here are predecisions to be resolved by a "dress rehearsal" with the family: who drives you to the hospital and the best route without much traffic. Then check all the medical possibilities and capabilities in the area and how they can be reached in an emergency.

Modify and change behavioral habits. Most stress is self-inflicted, so analyze yourself. Make a list, heading it *Life and Death Habits to Practice.* Post it so your family can add a great deal more to the list. Make notes of excitements, your business drive, your rush to keep dates on time, other people's weaknesses that upset you, how to allow yourself more leeway time. Don't be impatient, hostile or aggressive. Pace yourself at weddings and funerals.

Travel changes. Before and after the time of travel are always critical. By planning well in advance each and every step throughout the trip, there will be no need to rush. Leave plenty of time for rest and relaxation whenever possible, and relieve stress with a tranquilizer if you think you need it.

The Bible tells us that "In the last days, perilous times

shall come and men shall be ever learning and never able to come to knowledge of the truth." I mention this because I know the problems. I had all sorts of trouble changing my character and disposition, and I occasionally falter in practicing what I am preaching. But I keep trying by knowing that a slip may result in my last heart attack. Practice, practice, practice.

HELP COMES IN PIECES

I am most indebted to my oldest son, Bob, for "tuning me in" on chelation therapy. Knowing only little about it at the time, I was telling friends jokingly that I was thinking about having an enema of the arteries instead of bypass surgery.

But as the information sifted in from various sources I began to gain confidence in the therapy. It was easy, inexpensive and evidently did a more thorough job than surgery. All I had to do is find out where I can receive such therapy.

And you will learn as I have, friends, that chelation therapy is a much better deal in all ways than bypass surgery. I have something that even the wealthy movie stars and politicians who have undergone bypass surgery cannot match now or possibly in the future. Lasting health, freedom from stress and worry, and happiness again. And thus, my heart attack was responsible for introducing me to an almost unknown medical therapy that could help many thousand of people as it helped me. Medical costs and suffering could be reduced in a revolutionary way.

I do not have to rely on the AMA non-endorsement of the therapy. I do not have to listen and decide about truth or fiction. My research paid off . . . for me.

But let's start at the batters box and let me take you around the bases slowly and hope, methodically, touching each base on this wonderful run to full health and vitality.

Just as your preventive physician takes you step by step in his holistic approach to health, each chapter of this book takes you closer to a new found way of life you are destined to enjoy.

SUMMARY THOUGHT!

Seeking a healthy heart in America may be like looking for healthy fish in a polluted stream. When we look at the causes always disputed, against the solutions, it seems we may be trying to upset a speeded-up sense of time built into our economic system.

Chapter Three

KILLER OF THE CENTURY

"Two great physicians first, my loving husband tried to ease my pain . . . in vain, at least he got a third, and then I died."
. . . Epitath in a Churchyard

HEART #1 ATTACK

Wake up America . . . your diet is dangerous to your health! Arteriosclerosis and its many miseries have reached epidemic proportions during the past 15 years. The "cure" for this has been under dispute for well over 20 years. The broad cause is widely accepted, blaming it on the food we eat. The narrowed-down cause, or more definite cause, is very slowly being resolved but still under dispute by conventional medicine. It is at this point I can recommend definite answers . . . backed by my own experience, that of the American Academy of Medical Preventics (AAMP), and many researchers, and the latest information on the subject.

If you are forty years old, chances are you have some degree of arteriosclerosis. It starts much earlier in life. The cause of this is the mushy, wax-like sticky mess built up between the walls of the arteries. As this "plaque" builds up the flow of blood is restricted, and nature must adjust itself to the gradual increasing problem. Eventually the arteries become stiff and hard; the build-up distorts their size and shape; the flow becomes more restricted and taxes the circulatory system. It is at this point that the body finds itself

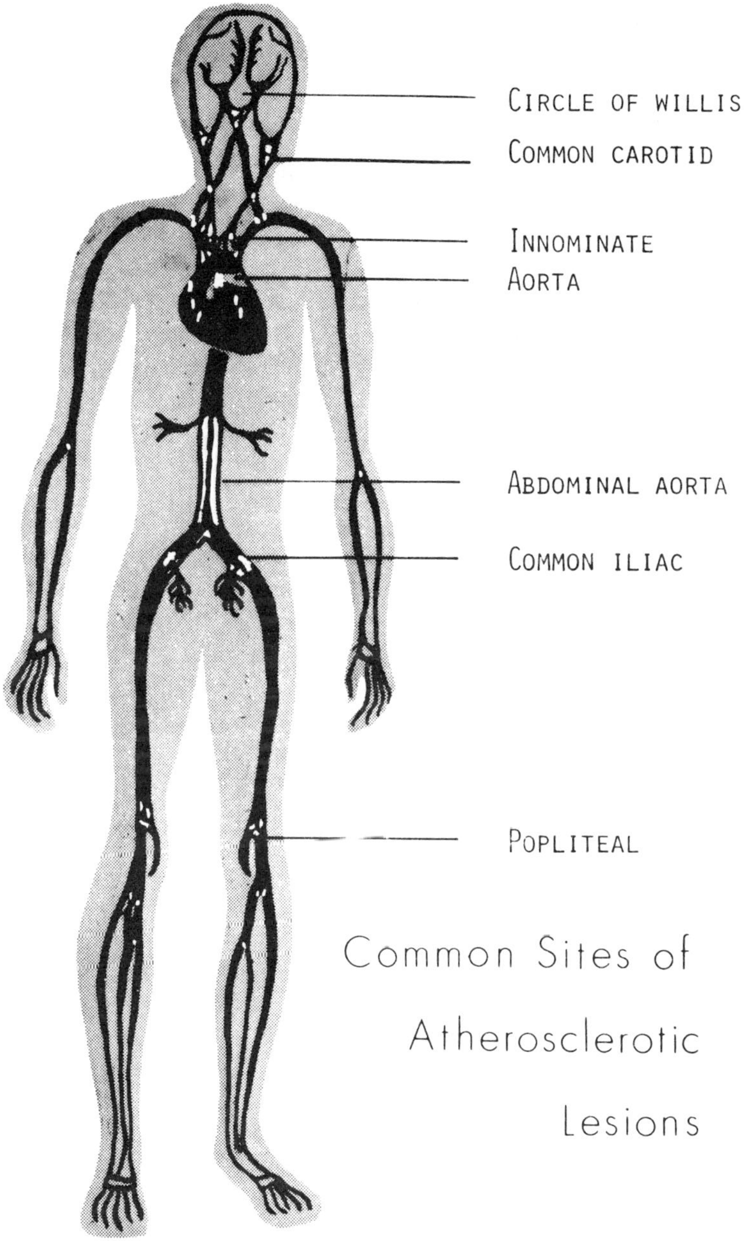

Common Sites of Atherosclerotic Lesions

hardly able to stand the abuse of its complex functions . . . high blood pressure, hypertension, angina pain, shortness of breath can occur. The "breaking point" of this bodily abuse is a heart attack.

The dispute I mentioned is over the *"cause"*. Those involved are in government with their protectionism (the Food and Drug Administration), the USDA (Dept. of Agriculture), the American Heart Association (who should know better), and the Food industry along with the Drug industry. These groups, along with the American Medical Association (AMA), have continuously blamed cholesterol as the cause. The 10,000 heart attacks every day in the United States seem to make them shout all the louder about cholesterol intake. No one seems to take time to "eat their words" or retract the facts, as their supporters are fed with ringing cash registers that help support their motives or thinking.

They tell you to cut out eggs. They are high in cholesterol. They sell "Egg Beaters," a man-made look-alike, as a substitute for this 'dangerous eating practice . This is just one example of the problem we have taken on ourselves from our eating habits and the food we are told to eat by the various media.

I have a report from the Burnside Research Laboratory[8] at the University of Illinois (Urbana, Illinois 61801). It is authored by Meena Kasmaii Navidi, M.S., and Fred A. Kummerow, Ph.D. It was reported from *Pediatrics,* Vol. 53, No. 4, April 1974. It concerns test comparisons of farm fresh eggs, "Egg Beaters" (the substitute), and a regular diet fed laboratory rats, called Purina Chow. There are nutrient values charged in the three categories. The two egg products were fairly close in some areas of comparisons; real eggs higher in value, the Chow as quite a bit better in nutritional value.

The photo reproduction you see shows the vast difference in the two egg products. The rats were weighed for comparisons in size before and after the studies. The "Egg Beaters" averaged 3.6 gr.; those fed whole eggs weighed 66.5 gr.; while the Chow rats averaged 70 gr., as a result of final tests. The actual report is much more startling, but the photo should suffice to show what can happen when we are misled. Four weeks later all the rats weaned on an egg substitute diet were dead.

If you could see inside random samples of arteries of

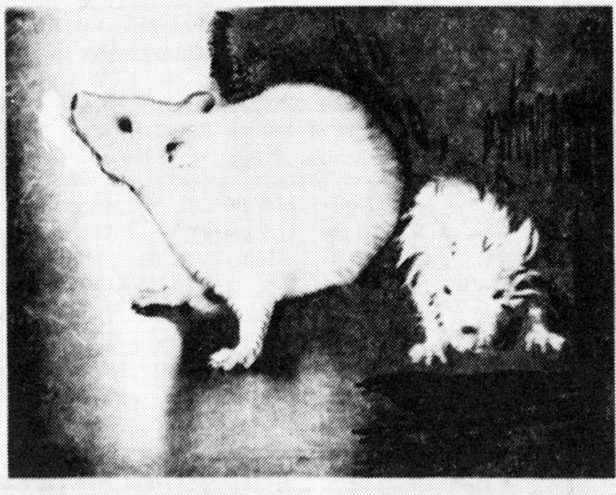

Weanling rats fed shell eggs (left) and Egg Beaters (right).

age groups from 20 to 60 years, as I have, it would make your hair curl. They appear as mountain ranges, craters and hills. You see the actual degradation of the inside of the arteries over the years . . . and wonder how they pass blood through at all. I am not speaking of arteries of sick people; they are average and taken close to the heart, during autopsies.

Here are some risk factors in what this plaque does to arteries and the effects to the body . . .

- It forms around the bone area of the ear causing head noises, ringing, and sometimes deafness.
- It collects in the gall bladder . . . forms gall stones.
- It collects in the body joints of the bones causing some types of arthritis.
- The lumps can break loose as the artery wall bursts or ruptures causing cerebral hemmorhage or stroke. The word is "aneurysm."
- It collects in the eye and can cause blindness. It can be seen by examination of the eye.
- It can cause problems in the prostate gland.
- It causes the age-old problem called "hardening of the arteries," a condition often apparent in the faces of older people.
- It causes senility with sometimes severe memory loss.

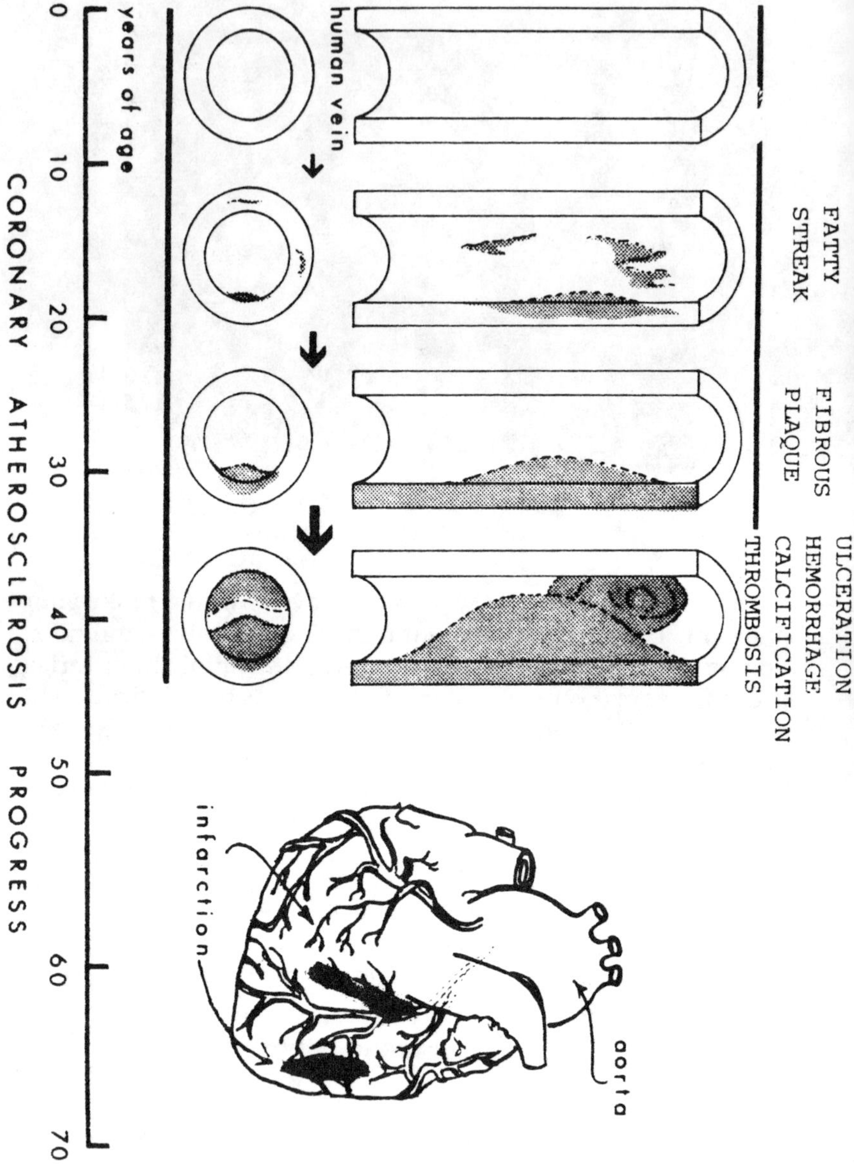

PROGRESSION OF ARTERY INVOLVEMENT

Schematic concept showing the progression with age of coronary atherosclerosis. Fatty streaks are found in early lesions which sometimes regress. Fibrous plaques progress to a point of complicated hemorrhage, ulceration, calcification, or thrombosis, that may produce myocardial infarction.

These arteries are reduced in size as our circulation is impaired, as we feel "cold feet" and "cold hands" at the extremities. The heart pumps harder just to "keep up" to the restrictions. Indicated usually by high blood pressure.

You may ask about cholesterol in the food we eat causing heart disease. This is part of the dispute and is not true. There are hundreds of studies and proof of this fact. Since cholesterol and fats are found in the plaques, the quick reasoning was that it was the proper identification of the entire problem, and we seem to be "stuck" with this improper hypothesis. The only accurate relationship is really *too many calories,* which is excess body fat. Richard Passwater, in *Supernutrition for Healthy Hearts,* is most emphatic and furnishes a world of proof that cholesterol does not cause heart disease; that dietary fat does *not* raise cholesterol levels; that eggs are good nutritional food.

Let's look a little further. There's a discovery of Dr. Earl Benditt of Univ. of Washington, School of Medicine, Seattle, that a group of identical cells growing from a single cell produces arteriosclerotic plaque. The last step in plaque formation is calcification. Once cholesterol has been produced within the fibrous plaque, the calcium is held to the plaque by an electrical charge, and the addition of calcium hardens the plaque. This plaque building continues as the calcium attracts more material from the blood stream . . . including cholesterol and triglicerides. The electrical charge makes the plaque grow layer by layer.

As you can see from drawings, these plaques form near junctions of the arteries. As plaque builds up it slows down the flow of blood and increases plaque formation at these restrictive junctions.

Calcium metabolism is important in understanding arteriosclerosis, aging, and other degenerative diseases. More important, calcium removal is the major objective in chelation therapy, which we will discuss in later chapters.

Calcium is the most dominant mineral in the body. It plays an important role in numerous cellular functions and has a pronounced effect on cell membranes. It is too extensive a subject to deal with by this layman. For instance, the bones of the body are made up of calcium in one form; the calcium in plaque is of another form . . . the form that is chemically removable by the infusion of EDTA by chelation therapy. One is not affected by the other. There is calcification in arteriosclerosis; there are dietary forms of calcium; and there is regulation of calcium "transport" . . . all dealing with the complicated metabolism of calcium.

Lifestyles are directly related to heart disease. There have been many studies on lifestyles as the cause of artery problems. In my own case, I mentioned my eating habits and activities as a salesman on the road. A study in California of 4000 Japanese-Americans indicated that lifestyle was more important than cholesterol and fat in the diet. The Japanese-Americans maintaining Japanese culture had lower rates of heart diseases than those Japanese-Americans who shifted to the American lifestyle.

Studies of various populations in the world having little or no heart disease have been completed many years ago. The Maasai of Tazania; Sweden, where heart disease rate is ⅔ that of the United States; the Eskimos' primitive living; the Benedictine Monks, all different studies showing diet and lifestyle, not cholesterol as the primary cause.

In short . . . the evidence is overwhelming that the cholesterol theory is not important in our living process.

Fortunately for mankind, the circulatory system has a built-in safety mechanism to withstand a certain amount of obstruction. The flow through the average vessel, I am told, is far greater than the organ it supplies really needs. In fact, it isn't until the diameter of the vessel is reduced 50 percent that significant change can be noted in the tissue it supplies, and even 70 percent reduction in flow is tolerated reasonably well.

This great margin of tolerance is what permits young people to function without symptoms of clinical heart disease, even though the process of arteriosclerosis, which starts early in childhood, has already produced measurable narrowing of the arteries. The many stress factors, nutritional defects, environmental poisons, etc., may accelerate the process so much that it no longer is unusual to see people in their forties struck down in their prime of life by a heart attact or stroke.

No one just developes a heart attack or stroke or a blood clot without a history of slow insidious build-up inside blood vessels. Until that fact is universally recognized, organized medicine will not advance beyond the symptom therapy stage. The great advance lies in preventive medicine and clearing the arteries of deposits which close them before the symptoms or attack, which makes the problem obvious to everyone. This is where chelation therapy has its greatest future, so say's William J. Goldwag, M.D., of Stanton, Calif.

Medical science, like the river, just keeps rolling along . . . a slow, never-ending process of medical breakthroughs though not yet fully accepted. Many years later the same breakthrough is rated confirmed, true, but of little use. Then, many years later, the breakthrough becomes a discovery of importance. Many times they take so long to become recognized as important discoveries that they are already outmoded by new breakthroughs. But let's go one step forward . . . instead of a breakthrough, let's call this book a "rediscovery".

Occlusive heart disease or arteriosclerosis is no longer considered an old man's disease. No longer should it be called degenerative (in most cases), but more like a "deteriorating condition" that can be cured without surgery. It is no longer necessary to be inefficent and decadent. There are answers. I am living proof that the cures are here *now, today.* They were discovered many years ago and are perfected . . . all we have to do is screw some heads on the right way, and we will all be most grateful.

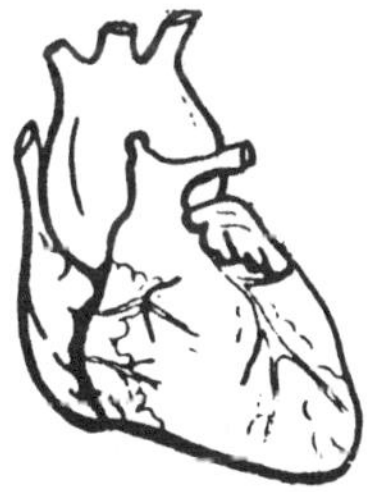

Good Circulation — Good Nutrition, The HEART of Good Health

SUMMARY THOUGHT!

There is a lot more involved in prolonging your life — there is MAKING LIFE WORTH LIVING.

Chapter Four
THE HEART ENDURES

"Those who bring sunshine to the lives of others cannot keep it from themselves."

. . . James Barrie

The heart is not a delicate organ. It is very tough. For months before birth, until death, the heart like the river, just keeps rolling along. It continues its rhythmic muscular contractions, relaxing for only a fraction of a second, and contracting again. This is an endurance task far beyond the capacity of our other body muscles.

The heart is normally strong and vigorous at fifty to sixty or at fifteen years. All other muscles will reach exhaustion from work or exercise long before the heart gives away.

Heart disease is not hereditary, although an hereditary tendency to heart problems is possible. This hereditary tendency can mentally predispose some people to heart disease, a different mental stress condition being the cause rather than inheriting the problem itself.

An interesting case of "over exertion" that ended happily in sports history was the Roger Bannister betterment of the four-minute mile record years ago. For *three hours* after that 3:58 minute record, this great English runner's pulse rate was 155 beats per minute, and finally slowed down. No doubt the delayed suffering had no permanent effect because of the training and physical condition of Bannister and his heart. It is an interesting example of what regular exercise can do for us.

The heart beats about 100,000 times a day and rests an equal number of times in between, but for a shorter period. The pump volume is about 4000 gallons of blood each day. The heart is like a variable volume pump in that it

The effects of exercise on heart action.

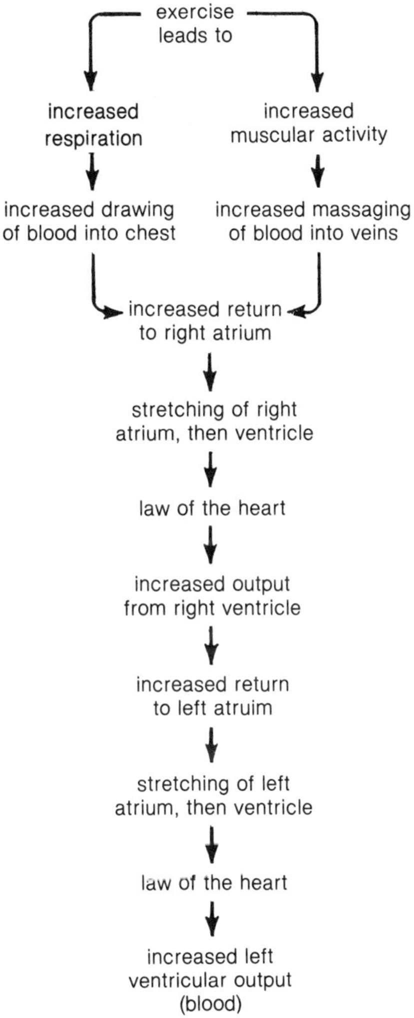

The effects of vasoconstriction on heart action.

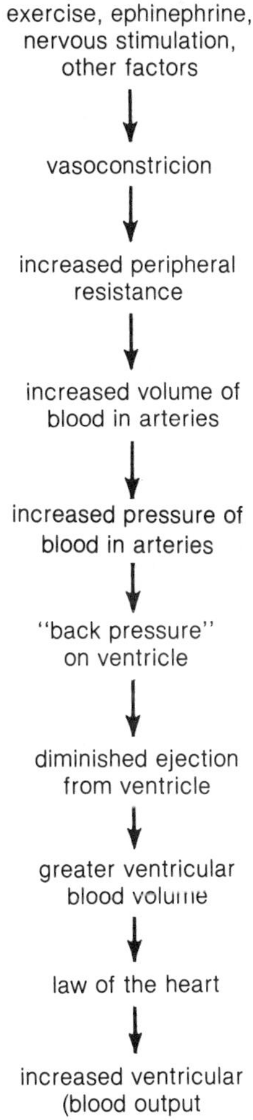

The vessels can change their diameter to a greater degree of their total diameter than any other vessel. A decrease in diameter (vasoconstriction) and an increase of diamter (vasodilation) increase and decrease peripheral resistance, respectively. Increased resistance calls for a greater pressure to maintain adequate flow through the narrowed channels.

can alter its output to the changing conditions put upon it. If you take the number of beats and multiply by the duration of the rest period (1/4 of a second) we have a total rest period of six hours per day. This is equal to about twenty years of rest in the average lifetime. Over a year's time the heart beats about 35,000,000 times. Imagine that in such an incredible organ, affected by good and bad influences, abused and misused by the food we feed it, the rest and exercise we give it, the heat and cold we subject it to and our everyday feelings and beliefs . . . our own mind's influence on it.

I don't know of any other machine on earth capable of working uninterrupted indefinitely without repairs; it has been said by scientists they believe this organ, with good care, can easily function for one hundred and forty years.

All the various mechanism govering the functioning of the heart, blood pressure, and blood flow are directed toward ensuring an ample supply of blood, nutrients and oxygen to the small EST capillaries where the vital exchanges of these gases, nutrients andwaste occur. Without these ingredients reaching the extremities, the tissue becomes dead and useless.

As the blood leaves the heart it is under extreme pump pressure. However, all the energy imparted to the blood by ventvicular contraction is not used in supporting the flow of blood. Some of this energy is used to expand the *elastic walls* of the large arteries. A movement or recoil of the arterial walls then assists the heart in pushing blood through the blood vessels. This wave of recoil is responsible for the *pulse wave* which can be felt in any artery close to the surface of the skin. The miracle of nature is, if these arteries were rigid instead of elastic tubes, with each heart beat the pressure would rise sharply in them but then fall sharply once the contraction was over. But blood flow is intermittent but rather still continuous, because of the elasticity of the arterial walls, so blood flow and blood pressure are easy to measure.

There are a number of regulators of arterial blood pressure all working in combination to maintain normal pressure. The pumping action of the heart; the elasticity of the arterial walls; the viscosity of the blood (thickness) and the peripheral resistance or arterioles (small arteries). So we can easily understand the harm done by these blockages.

Rapid adjustment of blood pressure is affected by the nervous mechanism controlling the heart rate, and the quality of the arterioles. The smooth muscle walls of the arterioles can be caused to contract or relax by nervous impulses (stress). As with the heart, there are two sets of nerves going to these muscles, nerves which emanate from the central nervous system. So frustration, pent-up feelings, anger, etc. make there presence felt. These nerves which regulate contriction and dialation of blood vessels are called vasomotor nerves. The stimulation of one set, the vasoconstrictor nerves, causes contraction of the muscles; stimulation of the vasodilator nerves relaxes the muscles. Consequently, if a *large number* of blood vessels are constricted, the pressure rises and, if a large number are dialated, the blood pressure falls. The excessive pressure causes gradual degenerative changes over a period of time and the arteries *lose their elasticity.* This is where hardening of the arteries got its name.

The amount and rate of blood flow to a particular organ are regulated by nervous and chemical factors. The chemical effect appears to be predeominant. When an organ is active, its rate of metabolism increases and more carbon dioxide is produced than when it is at rest. The excess carbon dioxide diffuses into the blood stream and causes *dilation* of the arterioles (small arteries) of the organ by direct action of the smooth muscle walls. With increased efficiency of the arterioles, more blood is delivered to the organ at a faster rate. That increased efficiency naturally affects our well being and health, as the life giving blood reaches the extremities.

Emotional states are just as taxing on the heart muscles as physical activity, because they are *sustained longer.* When exercise or physical effort tire a person, he usually stops and rests. But when worry and anger cause fatigue, most people unfortunately stop everything but the worry and the anger.

Here again the billions of nerve and tissue cells are quickly affected by the various kinds of food we eat; and our emotions, by our climate, altitude, and even gravity. You get the message; we are affected by everything we do, or experience.

As blood goes, so goes the life of the person or, as the

Bible says, "the life of the flesh is in the blood". Here is an interesting comparison and the resulting problems. Picture this:

The wellness of a healthy person is pictured by fast flowing, rapidly circulating fresh blood, flowing around every cell and in and out of every tissue . . . a perfect situation. But at the other extreme there is a lifeless body; circulation has stopped completely. At opposite poles of blood circulation are found the perfectly healthy and vigorous person and a life less body. Between these two extremmes of perfect wellness and death may be found all the diseases that affect human beings, and would also be found some degree of blood strangulation, some impairment or deviation from perfect blood circulation.

In short, *all sickness* seems directly or indirectly affected by interference with the flow of blood. Such "roadblocks" to good circulation always place a strain on heart action. This confirms the statement on the cover of this book, that, every second person who dies in this country each year does so as a result either directly or indirectly from degeneration of the arteries. There's no need to die prematurely. Death from most heart diseases of 95% preventable. The reversal of this clogging condition can easily be accomplished with or without pain or medication and without surgery.

Chronic fatigue brought on by overwork and/or on the job, and nervousness can affect many people who develop nervous tensions and frustrations. This is caused by poor circulation of blood to the brain and, is *not* as we so often hear, "all in the mind." Good circulation is basic and must be restored, just as in fainting. Nothing else will do the job. Fainting is usually caused by sudden shock draining blood from the brain. Fainting is usually cured by allowing gravity to send blood back to the brain. But, this blood draining process could be dangerous and in time deprive the brain of its normal nourishment, and oxygen in its blood supply, causing depression and other personality problems. So you see, the basic problem in this instance, is the shortage of blood to the brain; the same problem of course could be affecting any part of the body in the control of our health and well being.

In the human body the vast majority of cells cannot receive nutrients directly from the outside, nor eliminate waste directly to the outside. The circulatory system is the transport mechanism with its many blood vessels feeding every inch of the body. The blood transport medium feeds new life into every cell and takes away its waste with unending efficiency.

Percent of all Deaths due to Cardiovascular Diseases by Age United States 1977

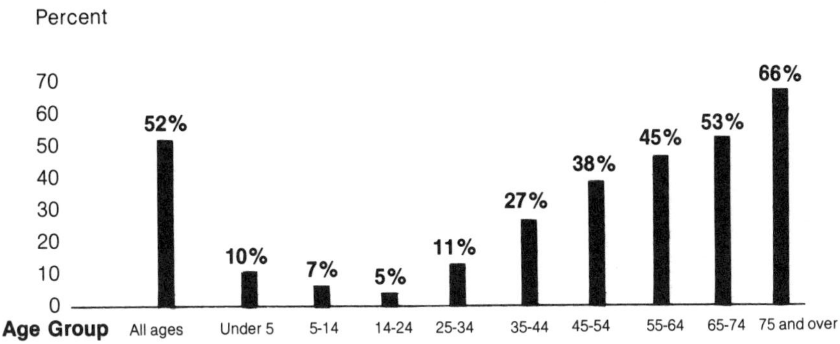

Source: National Center of Health Statistics U.S. Public Health Service HEW

Too much worldly striving, too little muscle activity, too little rest, bad food, smoking and drinking, all interfere with blood circulation. The resulting malnutrition of brain cells may reach a point that extreme nervousness, insomnia, or some hard-to-control emotional state may be experienced.

This inspires this writer to note that the durability of the heart is directly related to obstructions in the arteries developed over the years most slowly, to the eventual overtaxing of the heart to the point of no return. I found this out the hard way.

SUMMARY THOUGHT!

I know full well the moral significance . . . as the heart lives on as a pillar of strength and endurance, we are reminded of any injury we place upon it. Biological changes, resultant abuse, environment and stress make us mindful of the need to protect this organ as a major force in half our illnesses and in life itself.

Chapter Five

WHAT IS CHELATION THERAPY?

"I haven't heard of anyone who wants to stop living because of the cost."
. . . Frank McKinney Hubbard

Low cost, no risk, and the entire body of arteries cleansed, are three most favorable features of chelation therapy. This is exactly what sold me on this treatment. It is 1/15th to 1/25th the cost of major open-heart surgery, that only bypasses the problem area going into the heart. It is virtually risk-free. There has never been a death attributed directly to this therapy. Its also called endarterectomy. The "cleaning out" action works from head to toes, and refers to the removal of material from within an artery. The total reward starts with a new enthusiastic and fruitful "life is worth living" attitude.

The earliest literature on EDTA (ethylene diamine tetracetic acid) is dated 1937 where it started in Germany. EDTA was synthesized in the United States in 1933. Both United States and German patents were filed in 1941.

Various new discoveries on chelation therapy were reported in the Journal of the American Medical Association starting about 1950. After a period of three decades, more than 270,000 patients have received in excess of 4 million treatments in the United States alone.

The successful treatments for catastrophic effects of artery disease, stroke, senility, early gangrene, essential hypertension, peripheral vascular occlusive disease, osteoarthritis and related disorders have been administered by physicians for over 20 years. So we cannot call it a "new" therapy even though most people have never heard of it.

In addition, the results of chelation therapy treatments showed definite improvement in circulation of the patient as evidenced by improvement in skin color, arterial pulsation in the feet, a return to normal temperature to the feet, regaining the ability to walk long distances comfortably, improved brain function and important muscle coordination. The patient has no angina pain and no longer has to rely on the use of nitroglycerine, or various dilating drugs taken by heart disease victims.

In some cases, chelation therapy has been found to improve kidney function, remove environmental poisons, stress factors, air pollutants, heart valve calcification, digitalis intoxification, calcimosis, scherodema, empheysema, Parkinson's Disease, leg ulcers, significant improvement in arthritis, and it has also been known to decrease the amount of insulin required in diabetes.

Every cell and tissue of the body is dependent totally upon blood circulation to bring essential nutrients to it and carry away toxic products of metabolism. Any process that interferes with this constant flow will upset the delicate balance in the cell, change its ability to function properly, and allow it to fall prey to toxic and hostile elements in the environemnt of the cell of tissue, and, eventually result in disease. (See appendix 1)

Practically every enzyme in the body has some small amount of metal involved in its chemical structure. The metal is found in *chelated form*. Without the trace metal, the enzyme is inactive. So we see that chelation is a process vital to all our proper body functions and survival.

Every mineral taken into the body with food or supplements must be chelated by the body *before* it can be properly utilized. If not chelated or bound it will stay ionic, and in this form, if in excess, will end up forming a stone or a sclerosis. So we see that chelation, a chemical reaction, has always been a vital function in our bodies.

The word *chelate* comes from the Greek word *chele* meaning to claw (as in crab claw). It refers to certain metals that are bound to other molecules and proteins, that are able to *claw out* these metals from the chemical itself. If you are familiar with the word *sequester*, meaning to withdraw, pull out, or hold out, you see a chemical process that was used to cure lead poisoning in humans many years ago and is still the treatment used today for chelating lead out of our bodies. Chelation and EDTA the chemical itself in some applications of commerical chemistry is called a *sequestering agent.*

The chelate EDTA or disodium ethylenediamine tetraacetic acid, is a synthetic amino acid. It has the power to chemically bind itself to calcium and/other minerals. One molecule of EDTA can pick up and bind three molecules of calcium, a bargain deal. If you remember earlier I called its use "enema of the arteries," and that is almost how it is accomplished chemically, moving out finally by way of the liver and kidneys harmlessly. There are no redeposits in these organs. You might think of it as a plumber reaming out a half clogged pipe.

It is however purposely a very slow biochemical process carried in the bloodstream that grabs that calcium molecules formed in the hardened plague, loosing the accumulated fats and flushing them all out eventually by way of the urine and kidneys.

Is EDTA a safe chemical to use? Well it is used in many processed foods such as mayonnaise and salad dressing. Many amino acids are present in our diets and in our bodies. There are about twenty-four of them. They are needed by the body to help enzyme action in metabolism. Of the daily amounts of protein recommended for an adult, about 20 percent of the constituent amino acids should be the eight essential amino acids since these cannot be synthesized in adequate amounts by the body and must be present in out diet.

Vitamins C and E are chelating agents. They are components of enzyme molecules. The amino acid hystidine and cysteine are strong chelators. Other chelators are proteins like albumin, polypeptides, vitamin A, and nucleic acid, all of which are indispensable to life itself.

Cheltation is of vital importance to the successful drugs that depend on chelation processes. These include antobiotics such as penicillin, tetracylines, streptomycin, bacitracin, polymixin, insoniazid and amino salicylic acid. So we will soon be impressed with the meaning and the effects of chelation in many more ways than this particular therapy portrays.

Chelation is also a *natural* function that takes place within all living organisms, both plant and animal. It is a chemical means by which plants and animals are able to utilize the inorganic minerals. Chlorophyll, for instance, the green matter in plants, is a chelate of magnesium. Hemoglobin, the pigment that carries oxygen in the red blood cells, is a chelate of iron (remember Geritol and iron deficient anemia). Chelation is involved in the formation and function of enzymes, the important substances that control most all of our vital functions in the body.

If you purchase mineral supplements that should be chelates of the mineral, as minerals depend on chelates for reactions.

Chelation therapy when used for treatment on a patient is a simple infusion process. The EDTA is mixed with the sterile infusion material (there are several) for infusion into the arm or hand. All you feel is the initial small needle prick. The gradual drip process, that can be regulated, takes two to four hours to complete and is tailored to the patient's condition. Near the end of the "bag emptying" process a series of vitamins and minerals is added to the process itself to go directly into the blood stream.

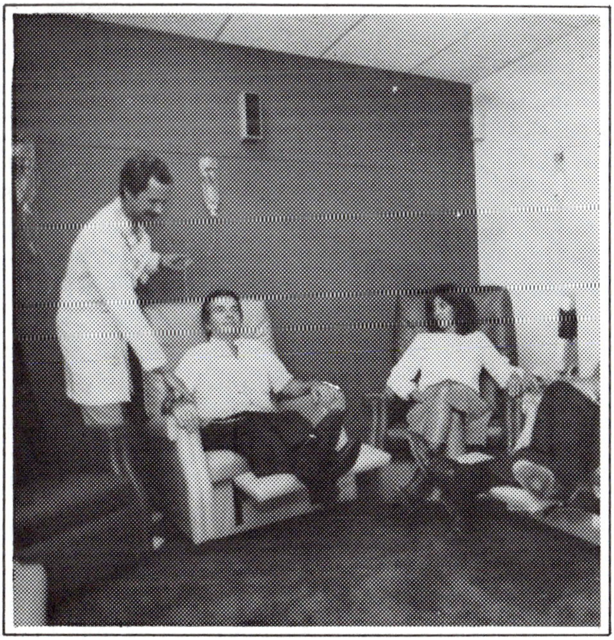

The atmosphere in the treatment rooms is rather unusual and one of neighborly informal, happy conversation, with patients sitting side by side or reclining in groups. You will hear many stories and helpful hints that will keep you better informed on your general well-being. Its a great place to learn from other victims.

The effects of chelation therapy may be dramatic in a short period of time, or it may take much longer.. Some people who could not walk across a room without angina pains were out playing golf in six or more weeks.

Treatments are usually given two or three times a week for a series of five to thirty or sometimes forty infusions. You, the patient, are the determining factor on continuance of the treatments. It is almost like a free trial (without the free). If you don't *feel* you are being helped — you can stop, but give it the benefit of your patience and reasoning.

As the mineral molecules are eliminated from the artery walls, they are washed from the bloodstream to the liver which then excretes it to the kidneys.

Dr. Norman E. Clarke, Sr., a cardiologist as the Providence Hospital in Detroit is "the" pioneer in this medical process. He observed, in a treatment of battery factory workers for lead poisoning, that the treated patients began to report alleviation of their symptoms of chest pains, claudication (pain in the large muscle of the leg due to lack of oxygen carried by the artery system), and an increase in the patients' well being and exercise tolerance. He is credited as having been the first to use it on human beings in this country. He is also hailed as a pioneer by the Soviet Union where chelation therapy is the second most common treatment for artery disease and used a great deal for prevention.

There are twenty-one different demonstrated or postulated effects of EDTA in the body. The scientific literature on chelation therapy is most extensive. More than 1700 articles have been printed in English alone. Yet what we often encounter, and what I encountered, as we visit the average cardiologist or family physician and ask about chelation therapy, we are told that there is no real evidence of the therapy's positive effects and that it *might* be toxic. Many of them really don't know about the therapy. Some, if they know, pretend not to know. This problem is discussed in later chapters.

TISSUE LAYERS OF BLOOD VESSELS

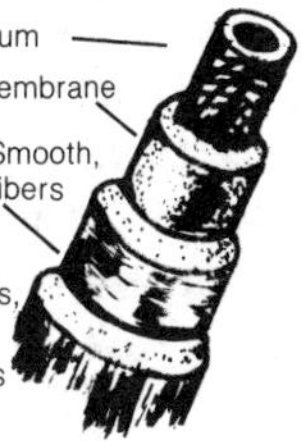

CROSS SECTION OF ARTERIES

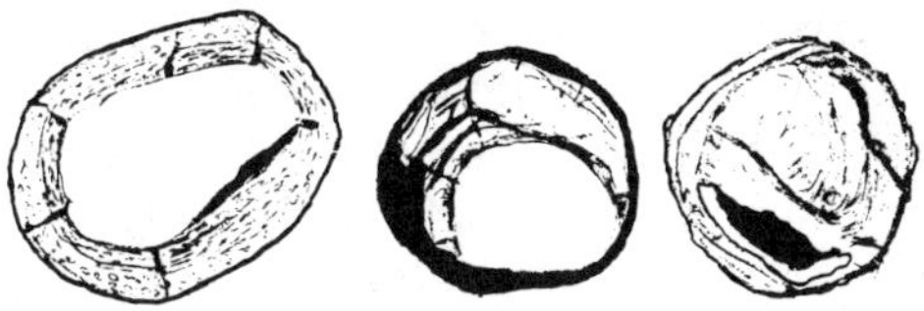

The deposits or plaque that accumulates in the arteries really forms within the intima, or inner layer, rather than the common notion of forming inside the artery surface. In advanced forms of arterosclerosis, the build-up finally erupts through the inner surface of the artery wall and the fatty build-up is exposed to the bloodstream where it does its damage.

Chelation therapy and EDTA attacks artheriosclerosis by acting primarily on the mineral content of diseased or occluded arteries. The major mineral is calcium, and as a person grows older, there is a slow progressive build-up of calcium in the cells of the body. These are mixed with fats, cholesterol and other matter forming a plague. Calcium deposition tends to impair the activity of the energy-related enzymes of the arterial wall. It also tends to harden the mixture like cement. EDTA removes some of the excessive cellular calcium of the arterial wall and helps to restore the normal enzyme functions.

Lipid peroxidation is a degenerative process that affects the cell in the arterial walls. EDTA assists by removing metallic particles in the wall membranes of the cell. These membranes, when destroyed, allow enzymes to escape and the cell is partially destroyed, EDTA and chelation protects this membrane by removing certain metallic particles that causes cell disease and destruction by peroxidation.

EDTA removes the "stickiness" of the blood platelets. Human blood consists of several elements: red blood cells, white blood cells, and platelets, all suspended in a complex liquid called plasma. The platelets' job is to repair small injuries or defects in the walls of blood vesels, this reduces hemorrage and promotes the clotting of blood. Under certain conditions these platelets become sticky and clot rather easily, and more than they should, This is a big problem in advanced artheriosclerosis and many types of heart disease, and may be life-threatening. EDTA tends to reduce the "stickiness" by removing the calcium from the platelets and thus *thins* the blood, So there is a two-fold benefit of EDTA.

The answer to a question frequently asked . . . calcium exists in the body in several forms which could affect the bones and teeth. But calcium is bound to protein and other molecules in a different way in the bones and teeth and *not* removed or affected by chelation action.

The most accessable forms of calcium are in various areas of the body where they have been abnormally deposited. Such areas as the inner walls of the arteries, in joints, around ligaments and tendons, in the kidneys, pancreas and beneath the skin. These abnormal calcium deposits are almost like those found in the blood, and these calcium deposits, called calcification, are removed in the chelation process. So you see why chelation does so many good things for the body that had been desecrated by various illnesses.

In addition, the blood vessel opening is enlarged, blood flow increases, and general circulation of more blood flow naturally means better circulation and an overall feeling of improvement. Picture a circle that is half closed in around its circumference, If this diameter is increased by half, the blood flow more than doubles.

It should be emphasized that not everyone feels this circulatory improvement so fast. Many times the arteries in the legs and feet are so blocked it is almost impossible to get EDTA to act effectively. While it worked with me, extensive walking during the therapy allowing flexibility of restriction finally eased the leg pains. So you can see exercise helps the chelation action. Sometimes the patient needs hyperbaric oxygen therapy for this problem, in combination with EDTA therapy.

Chelation and the effects of EDTA are somewhat of a mystery. Like aspirin, it works on many different areas but we don't really know why. We know EDTA captures heavy metals and calcium and that other areas of the body are affected in positive ways. For instance, angina pain can have a quick response, stroke paralysis can sometimes receive relief in days, blood fat levels, less insulin requirements, arithritis pain lessened and many more theraputic effects points to strong benefits we hardly understand.

I suppose this is the reason so many patients feel the good effects so soon into the treatments. Many improvements noticed rather quickly, after years of slow progressive oxygen robbing build-up.

In addition, the effect of chelation therapy is not limited to the improvement of the circulatory system, but it is enhanced by the nutritional effects of a program as outlined in forthcoming chapters. They must work together, thus, vaulable nutrients are able to get into areas of the body that were obstructed so long before, where blood flow was limited or stopped.

Side effects of chelation are really minor in nature in most cases. EDTA is non-toxic but occasionally a patient feels nausea; burning or stinging at the site of infusion, easily corrected by a heating pad or reducing the infusing rate; dermatitis; muscle spasms; or thromboplebitis in the legs. All these effects can be corrected by spacing the treatments out, by exercise, and tender loving care by the attendant nurse. Any reaction felt is usually caused by the correct effects going on. For instance, I started getting headaches halfway through the treatments, but only after about twenty treatments. This headache went away during the night's sleep. I believe the EDTA was getting through new areas inside my head that were partially restricted before. This resulted in my headache.

The reduced accumulations of plaque in the blood vessels can easily be proven by infra-red thermographs before and after treatments. There are other simple non-invasive tests that you can receive to show before and after conditions. But the best test of all is your own feeling of well-being.

At present, oral chelation by EDTA is NOT available or satisfactory because it is so poorly absorbed into the system. This indirect method would require large doses to arrive at the effective dose in the right places. Perhaps an effective oral method will be forthcoming in the future. We may see calcium blockers come on the scene, before this oral method.

Although chelation is commonly used as a therapeutic therapy, it is most effective as a prevention measure if we are wise. With chelation, it is possible to prevent some of the more serious catastrophic events associated with occulsive heart disease. In short, an ounce of chelation prevention is much better than a pound of chelation cure, and less expensive in the long run.

IN SUMMARY . . . Many practicing conventional medicine will have you believe that chelation therapy is pure quackery. Others use scare tactics with the examples they use to quell questioners; others will say they don't know anything about the therapy, making it seem like it is strange or unpopular.

My attempt at honest, experienced reporting is to keep away from the technical part of the explanation while being convincing in my enthusiasm for helping others with the same problem. As you will read on you will learn much more that you will be privileged to read in print for the first time. But after finishing this book and you still have doubts or need additional proof, it is available. See the back of the book for ordering information. But please do not ask your present doctor about chelation; you may not receive the information you so richly deserve.

SUMMARY THOUGHT!

The successful supression of this medical technique for over twenty years, gives credence to the power of the AMA . . . Overcoming this suppressive force takes the power of the people.

Chapter Six

CHELATION THERAPY'S CORRECTION OF BIOLOGICAL AGING

"Tact is the art of making a point without making an enemy."
. . . Anon.

(A condensation of a paper by Donald G. Carpenter, Ph.D., published in the June 1980 issue of **Rejuvenation,** *and of an invited talk by him to the Atlanta, Georgia, May 1981 meeting of the American Academy of Medical Preventics.)*

In 90 percent of the cases, death due to arteriosclerosis-produced vascular insufficiency is now avoidable. Clinical evidence reveals that dangerous vascular deposits can be and are being removed by chelation therapy. For far more than demographic reasons, the significance of this is enormous.

The success of chelation therapy in treating vascular disease provides classic proof of the validity of the crosslinkage, diffusion, free radical and excess product theories of biological aging.

The integrated theory of aging (displayed in the accompanying illustration) reveals that there are four basic causes of biological aging — crosslinkagage, disproportionate growth, excess product accumulation, and the molecular damage categorized as dissociations, vacancies and replacements. Two composite theories incorporating the foregoing four are diffusion theory and mutation theory. Two theories which reveal amplification effects on biological aging are the cybernetic theory and immunologic theory.

Crosslinkage theory holds that biological aging is caused by gradually-increasing crosslinkage (the joining of

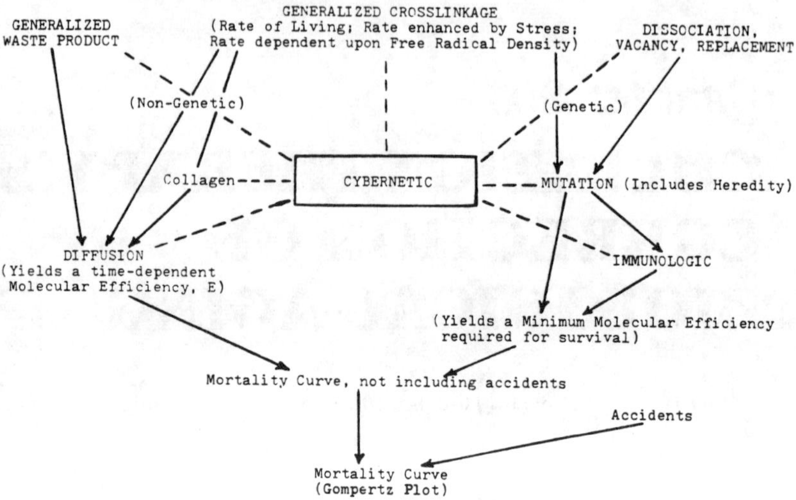

FIGURE 1. The Integrated Theory of Aging---- Flow Chart.[C4] The Cybernetic effect amplifies all of the other aging effects, its control and feedback actions are symbolized by the dashed lines.

molecules that do not bond together) in the body. This crosslinkage occurs both to non-genetic and genetic molecules. Minerals (such as calcium) are merely one type of crosslinkage-inducing agent. There are many types of such agents; calcium is the most important among the minerals.

Excess product theory holds that the accumulation of excess products (such as fats, sugars, waste products from you body's cells, and other such material) clogs and poisons your body. It blocks the flow of needed nutrients, stiffens membranes, and holds poisons in your body. It causes you to gradually weaken and to die.

Disproportionate growth occurs in such parts of your body as your connective tissue (collagen), the layers of your cornea, and your prostate (if you are a man). The extra tissue interferes with nutrient flow in, waste flow out, and with flexibility. Basically, such tissue as the collagen in your body continues to grow slowly after you reach adulthood; eventually it interferes with your health and well-being.

Dissociations, vacancies and replacements are produced in molecules by such things as transcription errors (during molecular production), external radiation, internal nuclear decay, quantum mechanical processes, etc.

Mutation theory holds that damage to genetic material produces mutations which accumulate and eventually cause system failure. (Note: Radiation and mutations account for perhaps 5 percent of biological aging.)

Diffusion theory proposes that some molecules are produced in your body faster than they can diffuse out; thus, they accumulate. Accumulation, crosslinkage and disproportionate growth decrease the diffusion coefficients to where you poison yourself while starving for nutrients.

Immunologic theory holds that mutations induce immunologic reactions with which you destroy yourself (arthritis, etc.).

Cybernetic theory points out that you are a feedback control system. The biological aging of your feedback controls (neurological, biochemical, biophysical) causes amplification of all effects of biological aging. For example, as crosslinkage, excess product accumulation and disproportionate growth interfere progressively with the flow of nutrients and consequently slow your metabolic rate; your body temperature lowers because of less heat production; the lowering of your temperature causes your neurological signals to become weaker and to move more slowly. Your physiological response to challenges (psychological, chemical or physical) therefore becomes less prompt and less adequate.

The importance here of the foregoing gerontological theories is their clarification of what is transpiring in diseases of vascular insufficiency, and of why chelation therapy is effective in coping with those diseases.

The genesis of vascular disease is composed of three stages. The first stage often involves a mutation (mutation theory) to the smooth muscle cells within the vascular wall. The mutation expands as a tumorlike growth into the bloodstream, interfering with bloodflow. The interior of the tumorlike growth often accumulates fats, cholesterol and other excess products (excess product theory) plaque build-up while mutated cells decay there.

In the second stage, turbulence around the tumorlike growth causes *excess products* to accumulate on the vascular wall (excess product theory). A blood clot also might form downstream of the growth and can actually exceed the original growth in size. Whether or not such a growth is present, excess product accretion tends to occur in any zone of turbulence — at valves, at branching locations, and at any location where the vascular lining is damaged or irritated. Such damage or irritation can be caused by carcinogens, allergens, refined sugar, physical stress, etc.

In the third stage, crosslinkage (usually with calcium as the crosslinkage agent) occurs, cementing the accretion/plaque in place (crosslinkage theory).

The deadly result is a gradual build-up of a chemical cement (called plaque) within your blood vessels. When a surgeon saws through a vein or artery which is impacted with arteriosclerotic cement, it sounds as if he is sawing through sheet metal. The growing blockage of cement slowly starves your body cells and causes poisons to accumulate within them. As if that isn't enough, think how long it takes the fat from a piece of warm meat to go rancid (not very long!). Then consider that the crosslinked fat trapped in your body has been there in some cases for many years; "rancid" might not be a strong enough word to describe it!

Excess product accumulation and crosslinkage (through vascular insufficiency) account for at least 50 percent of the deaths which occur each year . . . not counting the human suffering.

The fantastic news is that at least 90 percent of those deaths can be prevented. More than that, the health and vitality of those sufferers can be restored.

There is no secret as to how to reverse arteriosclerosis/angina/hypertensive heart disease, or any other disease of vascular insufficiency (ischemic heart disease/chronic disease of the endocardium/myocardial insufficiency and infarction/hypertension/some aspects of diabetes mellitus/etc.) The reversal is accomplished by chelation therapy. The chemical chelate removes the minerals (mostly calcium) from your blood. Your body produces its own chelate in an attempt to restore the normal calcium level of your blood. The combination of chelates de-cements the lining of your blood vessels; the sodium heparin in the chelate bottle dissolves blood clots; the vitamin C and stomach acid in the solution dissolve the rancid fats and other soft debris left on the vascular lining.

During the first ten sessions or so, the release of rancid fats and poisons usually results in nausea.

40

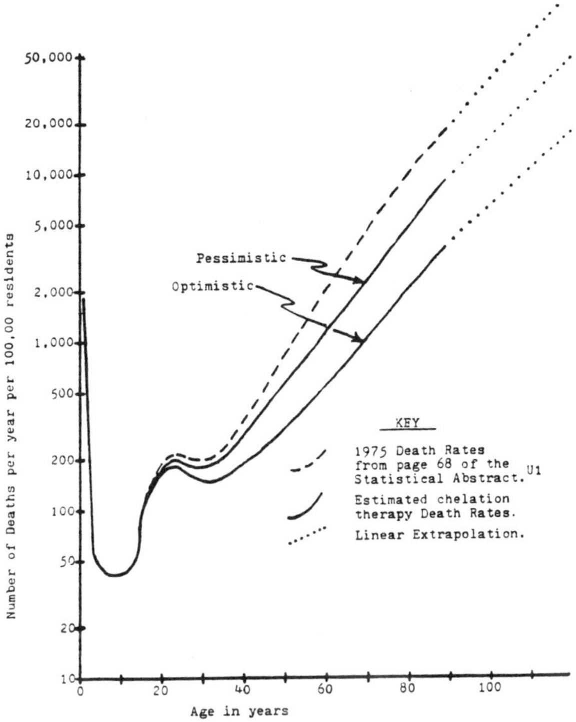

FIGURE 2. Male death rates by age. Estimated chelation therapy death rates are drawn from data in Tables 1 and 2.

But the end result is well worth the discomfort. Not only is there a 90 percent chance that your disease of vacular insufficiency will be cured (and the other ten percent might consist primarily of individuals who quit before taking enough bottles of chelate) but also your health and vitality will be so greatly improved that you will live in a lively fashion for many years more . . . and look younger too. A general rule of thumb is that a cure takes one bottle of chelate for each year of your life (more for some people, less for others).

The four basic causes of biological aging result in three types of clinical causes of death. 1. diseases of VI (vascular insufficiency), 2. malignancies, and 3. infections. Example of the three types of clinical causes of death are shown in the Male Death Rates illustration, as is an example of the fourth type (which is due to essentially random factors, although Maturation, depression and failing abilities due to biological aging do modify the otherwise random rate.)

Note that those clinical causes of death which are due to biological aging are steep lines on the semi-logarithmic plot. That means that biological aging death rates are essentially exponential.

The sum of all death rates by age is shown as a dashed line in the Corrected Death Rates illustration.

Chelation Therapy will essentially eliminate diseases of vascular insufficiency but the remaining random factors, malignancies and infections should yield total death rates in the neighborhood of the pessimistic and optimistic ones displayed.

It must be emphasized that the primary purpose of gerontologocal research is not to extend life but, rather, to reduce the pain and misery caused by biological aging. Because there is no quantitative measure available for pain and misery, we are forced to use the extension of lifespan as a measure of success.

The Anticipated Longetivity illustration (Male, the female illustration is similar and deleted) reveal the anticipated impact of chelation therapy upon mean lifespan.

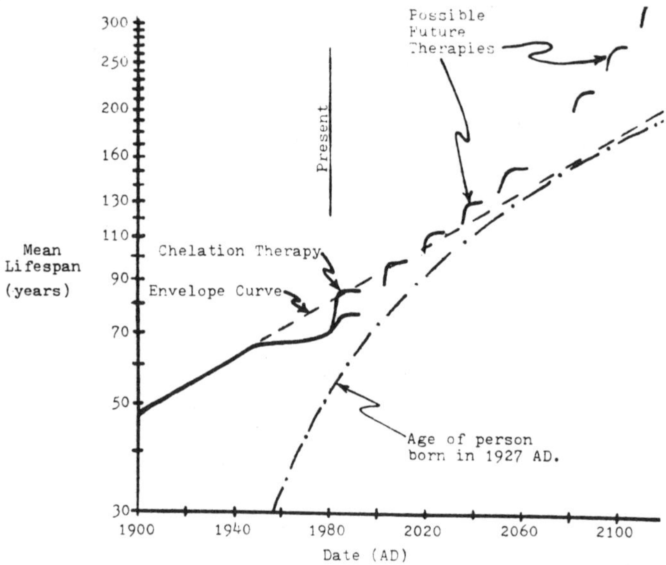

ANTICIPATED LONGEVITY VERSUS DATE (MALES)

And the dashed line is a technological forecasting tool which yields a conservative estimate of future achievements.

A man born in AD 1927 has approximately a 50-50 chance of survival past the year AD 2030. After AD 2030 he will become progressively younger physiologically until he becomes and remains physically in this twenties for his entire life. A woman born in AD 1927 has an even better chance of survival and recovery of youth.

Remember, though, that random factors (auto accidents, etc.) will probably keep the mean lifespan restricted to less than one or two hundred years.

In the United States, the birth rate has fallen below the replacement level for the population. That fact, and the fact that a longer life span enables greater knowledge, stability and productivity to be achieved by each individual, suggests that the correction of the basic causes of biological aging is occurring barely in time.

(See back pages in this book for availability of this paper in full detail.)

SUMMARY THOUGHT!

There is more to old age than something to exploit; there is respect. This type of medical care has grown at a faster rate for the aged than for anyone else. It now consumes 30 percent of our whole $200 billion medical bill.

Chapter Seven

BRAIN DISORDERS AND CHELATION THERAPY

"There is no such thing as incurable; there are only things for which man has not found a cure."

. . . Bernard Baruch

Conventional medicine has little to offer patients with brain disorders which includes cerebrovascular disease. Protracted morbidity, memory loss, confusion, personality changes, suicide tendencies, senility, are some of the symptoms.

Because brain disease is one of the leading incurable problems in this country, this chapter gains importance. But possibly more important is a cure for the suffering living, with old age and schitzophrenic symptoms. Chelation therapy takes on added importance since conventional medicine offers little help.

There has been little information to date on brain disease and the therapy for psychological relief by chelation therapy. You are receiving fresh news of proof of its effectiveness. The resulting vasodilation is considered a major breakthrough by those administering physicians who have experienced these remarkable results. Unfortunately such accomplishments in such a small group of physicians participating in these experiences adds little emphasis to the world of medicine, politics or to the general public.

The same sequence of events (plaque build up) that occurs in other organs of the body and extremities occur also in the arteries to the brain. Chelation therapy thus causes arteries to dilate and enhance blood flow to various parts of the body, including the brain.

We further learn that toxic metal poisoning can effect senility, and other brain disorders as we will find out as we read on. But let's look at the latest research . . . .

Dr. Lloyd Grumbles of Philadelphia presented a paper to the 1980 seminar of the American Academy of Medical Preventics in Chicago. Dr. Grumbles research showed remarkable help given to 20 patients where he administered chelation therapy and backed the treatments with before and after radioactive blood flow studies with the help of a computer. It was the first study of this nature which fortifies the progress of a series of chelation treatments.

Each patient was examined thoroughly before any treatments. There were twenty patients involved. All but one showed improvement in cerebral blood flow and all showed improvement in their mental or physical well being.

The one showing no improvement was almost a life-long schizophrenic, sixty years of age, a severe diabetic, smoker with an atrocious appetite. She panicked at the mention of insulin and there was no cooperation by the patient for any sort of treatment at all.

During the treatments Dr. Grumbles remarked that the patient became more open about her symptoms, which she had not been able to talk about before. She had been hallucinating since age seven. During that time she thought she heard voices coming from the walls and speaking foreign langugages. A language she would not think of using. Near the end of the treatment, even though her blood supply test showed no improvement, her voices had receded until they only involved her at home. This relief of phychic pain after all these years said Dr. Grumbles showed remarkable results.

Other notable reports concerned a seventy-five year old lady who after only ten treatments was relieved of her depression. A suicide depressed man whose family literally forced him into treatments and to the Doctors office. One day while having a treatment he broke from his usual silence and admitted that he felt great that day.

The other cases Dr. Grumbles described were similiar to those already described in the chapter LIVING LASTING PROOF but those cases described by Dr. Grumbles also were backed by blood flow studies as described.

Dr. Grumbles mentioned a patient who had been on disability for two years after a heart attack. The patient had almost complete relief from angina after the first chelation treatment. While this in itself is unusual, after twenty treatments he went back to work full time. Most important is the fact that two physicians had examined this patient and certified that he was disabled and unable to perform any work, in order for him to be approved for medicare payments.

In summary Dr. Grumbles reported that nineteen of the twenty patients showed universal improvement in blood flow to the brain as well as mental and physical improvement. The schizophrenic lady patient showed no improvement in blood flow but had a remarkable change in character.

Dr. Grumbles remarked that he hoped from this study to convince the public, a few cardiologist's, insurance companies and even Medicare that it was less expensive to spend one-tenth as much money on chelation therapy, that it was for all practical purposes harmless as compared to the appalling results from bypass surgery.

The use of megavitamin therapy added to chelation therapy, of patients suffering from schizophrenia and other brain function problems, helps reduce the need for drugs that are usually used in this treatment. Megavitamin therapy reduces the need of the drugs and protects against the harmful side effects of the drugs as well. The patient is spared much expense and doctor visits are reduced considerably. As related above, marked improvement resulting from chelation therapy is the first sign of progress in brain problems. Megavitamin therapy gradually reduces the need for drugs and the expense of visits to doctors and hospitals.

Teaching a patient to cope with stress or shock, or attempting to cure him by drugs will not alleviate the underlying problem of malnutrition, genetic defect, or circulation problem. You have to treat all the underlying problems.

The effect of brain problems and the resulting help given by chelation therapy and proper nutrition bring arguments from conventional medicine who treat the conditions with drugs that are mainly suppressive in nature. But the very least chelation therapy could do would be to lessen the intake of prescribed drugs. Particularly since most patients are rendered incompetent, senseless, feeble or dotish, they leave much to be desired as drugs just stabilize the patient.

H. Richard Casdorph, M.D. Ph.D. has recently released a paper EDTA CHELATION THERAPY II, EFFICACY IN BRAIN DISORDERS. The paper published in the Fall Edition of THE JOURNAL OF HOLISTIC MEDICINE, 1981, Vol. 3 #2.

Dr. Casdorph presented this paper as a result of the objective measurement of patients improvemennt resulting from intraveinous treatment of EDTA. The first time reporting is similar to Dr. Grumbles work just described but scientifically complete.

The study reported was performed in the Nuclear Medicine Department of Long Beach (Calif) Community Hospital. The scintillation camera is attached to a microprocessor and the data recorded on floppy discs.

The patients were positioned with the scintillation crystal assembly suspended above the patients head. Twenty millicuries of Technetium 99m were injected into the vein and blood flow was recorded. By computer reconstruction, blood flow to the sides of the brain were displayed and printed out.

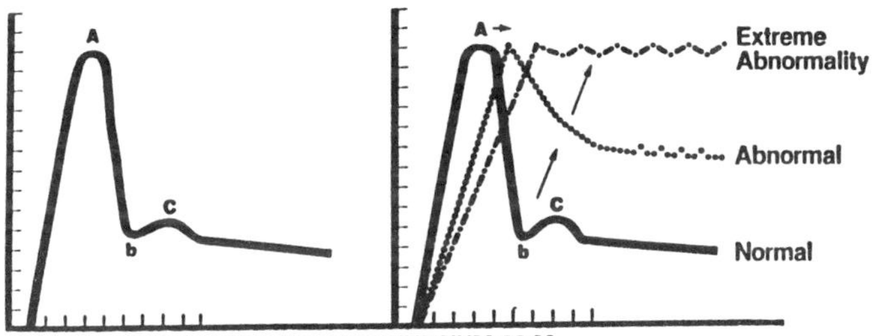

BRAIN FLOW STUDIES WITH TECHNETIUM 99 M.

Of the fifteen patients involved in the tests, their ages ranged from 51 years to 92 years. The number of chelation treatments given ranged from 13 to 20. They were male and female. There is a recorded chart on each patient with right and left side on the brain recorded before and after the treatments.

The advantages of these studies is that each patient serves as his or her own control, making marked results highly significant and statistically significant.

A variety of diagnosis of these tested patients consisted of cerebral atrophy with dilusions and hallucinations, without family recognition and with contemplation of institutionalizing. Documented schizophrenia, transient cerebral ischemic attacks, cerebrovascular accident and Alzheimers Disease were some the patient problems.

The result of the report is technical in nature and much more complete than this brief description. Each individual chart on each patient completed before and after chelation therapy were compared by the brain wave recordings. Such measurements of these charts showed a 71 percent return toward normal in comparative charts. Without a doubt a most impressive and noteworthy accompishment.

As Dr. Casdorph remarked, "This study is especially noteworthy in view of the fact that medical science has no effective treatment for many of these conditions."

Reported at the same Chicago seminar was added member documentation and discussion of phycological problems and treatment with chelation therapy. This problem of senility, unjustly called an old age disease, can be treated and relieved in many cases with the use of food supplements, to rectify the basic problem of chemical imbalance caused by restricted circulation to the brain.

A pioneer in chelation therapy, author of many books and lecturer, Dr. Bruce Halstead, was a featured speaker on brain disorders.

Dr. Halstead said that he now combines chelation therapy with hyperbaric oxygen therapy for improved results in cases of depression, memory loss and associated symptoms.

Hypernbaric oxygen therapy has been used by the Navy and Air Force for decompression sickness primarily in various veteran hospitals. It consists of forcing pure doses of oxygen into the body for absorption in the body. to help activate the body chemistry, stunt free radicals and other complicated functions. It is another area of help in preventive medicine that is gaining acceptance fast, to help formulate a cure rather than ordinary stabilizing medical treatment we all have been so used to in conventional medicine.

Dr. Halstead relates one particular success story something like this: At age five this boy played Bach and Beethoven on this violin. At age seventeen he played in the Boston Symphony Orchestra. At age thirty-seven he retired from a very lucrative real estate business. Whereupon he grew restless. In such a boring life he began practicing law.

At age seventy-three his problems were almost insurmountable. He had enormous loss of memory, was almost completely incoherent and was turning into a vergetable. His loyal and loving wife made the rounds with him to famous hospitals and clinics and he was examined by neurologists, psychiatrists, physicians and neurosurgeons. Money was no object in the pursuit of a cure or even a little help, as his wife continued to seek any help she could find.

Finally she heard or read about chelation therapy, and discussed her husband's problems with Dr. Halstead. Upon being fairly convinced that chelation would possibly help, and with no guarantees, she discussed the feasibility of chelation therapy treatments with the same previous brain specialists. Upon hearing her story, these physicians told the woman that chelation was sheer quackery. That if she insisted of going ahead with chelation treatments, it really could do no harm except possibly to his kidneys. That all the damage was already done on her husband, so a little more would hardly matter.

When Dr. Halstead examined this man initially his eyes were glassy as he was described as "looking through you". There was no intelligent conversation. A completely helpless individual led around like a dog on a leash. He was treated with forty chelation treatments and a like number of hyperbaric oxygen therapy treatments.

One month before the presidential elections he was explaining to his wife about Jimmy Carter and about his little known problems in politics. To read and make such serious analysis and statements Dr. Halstead said, was not done by a decrepit old man.

Two years later he was playing the violin and reading his law books again. His wife told of his interest in the "pretty gal" (nurse) who had been attending to him through the years.

NOTE: See ordering information in the rear of this book for complete availability of this and other scientific papers.

SUMMARY THOUGHT!

Paranoia, brain disorders or whatever madness is deeply rooted in our own problems of lifestyle, social and sexual equality. Like violence, seems deeply rooted in junk foods and the same equalities.

Chapter Eight
LIVING LASTING PROOF

"To his physician who said, 'General, I fear the angels are waiting for you'; 'Waiting are they? . . . Waiting are they? Well . . . let them wait'."

. . . Ethan Allen

The chelation therapy tecnique is condemned somewhat by the American Medical Association, whose August membership prefers the higher priced bypass surgery, although the difficult debilitating heart surgery cannot compare to the phenomenal **overall effects** of chelation therapy. Officially it is not approved by the FDA.

A report by a writer for the *National Tattler* narrates a typical incident. George M., age 54, was stricken with a heart attack in 1965. He flew to the famous Houston Clinic of Dr. Michael De Backy, internationally-famous heart specialist. After the routine tests that lasted five days, Dr. De Backy told Mr. M. , "We know what you have, but we don't know how you got it, and don't know how to get rid of it. There's a general build-up of deposits around the heart and there's no place to cut; therefore we cannot help you."

Mr. M. said he was "put out to pasture" by other doctors who attended him, and put on a low cholesterol diet and heart medicine. He said he barely existed for three years in pain.

After nine days of chelation therapy, Mr. M. noted a dramatic improvement and remarked that he felt like a new man again.

Because of the publicity from this newspaper article, there was tremendous response from readers, perhaps more than at any time in the publication's history. The paper discussed the many cures of chelation therapy and mentioned that it prevents heart attacks. These claims motivated the AMA to prosecute the doctor involved as a "quack" in spite of documented successful histories. California's health care authorities (CMA) become convinced that the AMA's claims of quackery were justified, and placed charges against the doctor. It went to court in 1974. According to the newspaper, the case was thrown out when the doctor and more than 900 patients prepared to prove the effectiveness of the therapy.

Then there was Sue who on her last birthday was 57 years old. She celebrated that birthday in 1976 in bed too tired to move. Sue said she was just waiting to die since doctors said that there was nothing that could be done for her, and that was her feelings then. Within twenty days of starting treatment she claimed was a miraculous therapeutic program, she noticed improved vision in her right eye, increased energy, and commented about the change in her appearance to her friends. There were no more blackouts, she could drive her car long distances, and began to attend dances every Friday and Saturday evenings.

Perry, a 70 year old retired military man, was an avid golfer until he lost so much energy he couldn't even play one hole, much less 18 holes. Walking was a task because of shortness of breath. He also had the problem of his right toe turning black and the nail dropping off. His feet were always cold. Within 20 treatments he had warm feet and was able to play golf again. He now plays 36 holes regularly when he isn't working eight hours a day, repairing old houses which he and his wife purchase for restoration.

Dr. F., M.D., of Long Beach, California, a popular Otolaryngolist was seized with severe chest pains while playing golf. He later visited his cardiologist and, following all the tests, the doctor was told he had obstructing plaque in the left main artery. They recommended a triple bypass operation. It must be done soon, his colleagues said, to avoid coronary occlusion and possibly sudden death.

Dr. F. was lucky . . . fate changed his course as the hospital could not find enough blood for his surgery until after the busy holiday season. During the wait, the doctor had the chance to discuss his problem with many colleagues and friends. He learned about a new therapy and began to search information on the subject. He was amazed to find *many medical journal articles on chelation therapy* for a treatment he had never heard of before.

He finally came east and entered the Alabama Hospital run by H. Ray Evers, M.D. Dr. F. remarked, he saw people come in with diabetic ulcerative lesions and gangrenous lesions that cleared up in 10 to 12 days. He said he witnessed a patient enter who was told his leg would have to be amputated because of gangrene. "I watched with my mouth agape as his leg came back to normal." Dr. F. was amazed that before, he could barely walk 10 to 15 steps without angina pain, but after 10 treatments the pain left completely. The doctor-patient has since given himself about eighty treatments with the aid of his nurse at home. He had not had an angina pain since 1972 . . . carries out a full day's workload plus 10 to 15 surgeries per week. He also swims 20 laps of his pool and plays golf regularly.

Talking about this pain (claudication), I used to wake up at nights with leg cramps they call "charlie horses." The only relief from these painful cramps was to rub the legs vigorously, stand up, and walk a little, unfortunately you were wide awake again.

This cramping was directly related to artery blockages, mainly in the leg. Chelation gradually opened the blockage; daily walking aided in stretching and better elasticity of the arteries; that in turn aided the chelation action. That activity could have built new collateral arteries in that area. I am not sure.

In 1973, Walter W. West had been suffering from severe angina pains. After a complete series of tests he was told that he had six months to a year to live without bypass surgery. He could not walk across the room without pain.

In 1975 he had a bypass operation and shortly thereafter complications, consisting of some angina, irregular heartbeat, fluid build-up and lung embolisms started. These medical problems forcd West to take disability retirement while he was still in his early fifties.

In 1979, West had a femoral bypass in the right leg so he would have some circulation in that leg. During early 1980 he had almost reverted back to his pre-bypass surgery status; poor circulation, angina pains, and almost a complete invalid . . . but with a new problem added, diabetes.

During the spring of 1980, having heard about chelation therapy, Walter West began treatments. He had to be driven on a four-hour ride each way, twice a week, for treatments. He now drives himself. He walks more than one mile each day, building up distance gradually. He is down from seven heart pills a day to just two, and he has had only twenty treatments. He has started reducing his insulin injections by five units per day.

Walter West was told at the Largo Clinic that he should be off insulin injections altogether by the time he has had thirty chelation treatments. In addition, West says he has much more energy and his angina pains are gone. He is really looking forward to renewed interest in his well-being and enthusiasm for life again.

In 1969, John Baxter, age 40 of Tampa, Florida, had a heart attack. In fact, he died and was revived with shock treatments. The doctors did not think that John was going to pull through but he made it. In 15 days he was out of the intensive care department.

Upon discharge, his angina pain persisted and later he had a catheterization (cath test). This led him into triple bypass surgery. Immediately after the surgery he hemorrhaged and received 16 pints of blood. Later , phneumonia set in and he was back in intensive care for 29 days.

Baxter complained of constant pain after the surgery had healed completely. He needed help to walk and upon complaint many times, was told that the pain was all in his head.

With his persistent complaint of pain he had a second cath test to find out why. This cath test took six and one half hours. (my cath test lasted about twenty-five minutes). The catherer was inserted in both arms and it was found that all the previous bypass passages were blocked. (This is the delicate and sometimes dangerouus part of the cath test.)

In March 1971 it was suggested that he have a second bypass operation in order to relieve the perisitent pain. Among the group of examining doctors, Baxter said, the consensus was that there was only a ten percent chance of getting off the operating table. But as a last resort, this surgery was performed and there was an improvement over the first operation, but the pain was only relieved; it did not stop completely.

In 1974, frustrated and pain ridden, Baxter decided to risk a trip to the Texas Heart Institute made famous by Doctor's Michael De Backy and Denton Cooley. A third cath test there showed an abundance of calcium build-up in the chest wall, and he was advised by Dr. Cooley that another operation would mean certain death. At this time in the story Baxter was taking 380 milligrams of Inderal per day. (I took 80 mg a day.)

During the next four years Mr. Baxter was in and out of the hospital with heart attacks and for emergency treatment of angina pains so severe he needed extra drug relief. He was a complete invalid, unable even to go to the bathroom.

The Baxter family heard at this time of Dr. Ray Evers clinic in Montgomery, Alabama. Against his better judgment and family insistance, he was driven up to the clinic by his wife. Under the worse medical conditions, his wife said, the hectic delays and urging to turn back by her husband somehow told her to keep going. Baxter had given up hope and considered the trip a worthless last resort.

Upon complete examination by Dr. Evers, Baxter was told that his chances of success were not at all good. This was his the worst case Dr. Evers had ever been involved with. But if Baxter was willing, he would give it a try with a series of chelation treatments.

Baxter had a treatment each day for three weeks. During this time he became discouraged as he was forced into all sorts of exercise programs and walking on a treadmill to a point of blisters and pain in the feet. But he persisted at the urging of his wife. At this point he began to feel better and encouraged. In five weeks he was jogging and ready to go home.

Baxter said that all told he had eleven heart attacks and four angina attacks requiring emergency hospital care. What he observed at the clinic was truly amazing, he remarked. For instance, a senility patient who was absolutely incoherent and in five to six weeks completely able to hold an intelligent conversation. Then there was the one-legged patient brought in with his other foot turned black with gangrene. With chelation therapy his foot had its natural color back and the patient was walking, able to put on a shoe and stocking.

As related elsewhere, Dr. Evers had been forced out of business by government harrassment and was in the Bahamas starting a clinic there. This was September of 1980 and Mr. Baxter received a series of twenty chelation treatments at a clinic operated by Dr. Donald Carrow.

Baxter now keeps active and out of his easy chair as much as possible. His gardening, odd jobs in remodeling for himself and his children keeps him busy. He said that he wants to keep active every day all day as well as his exercises. He says he sat in that chair too, too long and does not enjoy the chair anymore.

He is off all heart medication and does daily callisthenics including push-ups.

Baxter's final remarks are very noteworthy. He said he was very fortunate to have had good medical insurance and the he can get any sort of medical care as long as it is approved by AMA. Naturally, the medical treatments he has received and does not need anymore aggravate him. Why? The real irony of the situation is the only therapy he needs or wishes is chelation therapy . . . only he has to pay for it out of meager disability funds and it hurts his pocketbook. Since chelation therapy is not approved by the FDA. Medicare declines payment. Baxter says it is not only unjust but, like thousands of other disabled people, he would trade it all to be able to go back to work and a productive life again.

I wonder how many more disabled and medicare-paid individuals like Baxter have the same feeling. I wonder how many could be helped by chelation who have been put out to pasture needlessly. I wonder what this all costs us taxpayers . . . needlessly.

Lorene C., who lives in California was diagnosed as having advanced case of artherosclerosis. A school teacher who retired in 1973, she continued to tutor till gradually her energy was sapped to the point that after an hour of tutoring she was exhausted.

She spent most of her time in bed as she was overweight, (225 pounds). She had glaucoma, severe anemia, and continued to feel worse.

Through a health food store she heard of a lecture on chelation thereapy. Later she made a doctor appointment but felt so bad that she could barely answer the questions. "The doctor said that if I made it through fifteen treatments I would probably avoid a stroke. I started the therapy at once. And it brought me back to life, literally!"

Mrs. C. underwent 43 treatments before the calcium "really started being released". (There are measurements made.) She now walks five to seven miles a day, on hills. Her weight has dropped to 158 pounds. The glaucoma has cleared up, she says. Her memory is no longer foggy. In short "She's living again".

On one of her walks, she was stung by an insect on the leg. Infection set in and there was no doctors' offices opened till after the week-end, by Monday morning the leg was reddish black as she entered the doctor's office. He ordered a vitamin C infusion and told her that had it not been for the chelation treatments she may have lost her leg. Needless to say, Mrs. C. is not afraid to express herself on the merits of chelation therapy to anyone and as a witness, admonished the California Medical Quality Assurance Board for trying to stop the treatments in California.

FIRST HIS BROTHER

Another "believer" is Earnest, of Colton, California, who became a patient after he saw the transformation in his brother, Homer, of Arizona, whose heart stopped three minutes during an attack six years before, and was returned to life through electric shock.

"Ernie" as his friends call him, does not have a lot of extra cash . . . at 66 he lives prudently but comfortably with his wife on retirement income . . . so he wanted to be sure he was doing the right thing before he committed to the treatments.

"I waited until I saw how Homer came out before I started," he said "My brother had been told while in intensive care after a coronary, that there was nothing more they could do for him. So he just went home. He was so bad he just couldn't do anything. And when I went to see him after he had finished 20 treatments of chelation, he was working in the garden. And he also returned to work as a carpenter contractor. He was a different person!"

Earnest's first coronary was in 1962. Four years later he suffered a second one, and an angiogram showed that two coronary arteries were "totally blocked, and a third one was severely diseased". He was forced to quit his job as maintenance superintendent and endured severe angina pain from that time on.

The Appeals Judge, Tyrie Boyer, ruled against the Florida State Board of Medical Examiners, stating that, "they have no authority to deprive a doctor's patients from any therapy they wish. Just because most of the medical profession rejects certain treatments does not give the State Medical Board authority to punish a doctor for using it." He further stated, "history teaches us that virtually all progress in science and medicine has been accomplished as a result of courageous efforts of those members of the profession willing to pursue their theories in the face of tremendous odds and despite the criticism of fellow practitioners." Judge Boyer compared Dr. Rogers to Freud, Pasteur and Copernicus, as innovators in science and medicine.

The Florida Board of Medical Examiners, in order to save face, took Dr. Rogers favorable decision to the Florida Supreme Court for possible overturning of the appeal. In final disposition on September 8, 1980, Docket #56096, the six judges concurred with the appeals Judge Tyrie Boyer. The final text; "We hold that the boards' action is an unresonable exercise of the police power and we affirm the result of the District Court in quashing the order of the board." This sweeping and unprecedented decision means that doctors cannot be prohibited from using controversial treatments or drugs unless the measures have been proven harmful.

In reporting the decision, the *Brevard Today* newspaper I am told commented, that the opinion has far reaching implications . . . and that it could bring down an additional barrier to the use of laetrile, the controversial cancer drug, as well as other procedures and drugs that the medical profession calls quackery.

"God vindicates right and I believe we were right." commented Dr. Rogers. "There is always a danger of quackery, but that progress can only be achieved through new ideas."

The Florida Supreme Court agreed. "The record is replete with claimed instances of dramatic restoration of blood flow to the extremities resulting in arrest of gangrene, restored sensation, increased temperature and return of normal color to the toes, fingers, hands and feet after chelation therapy."

A victory for a faithful physician who perservered to the end. But also satisfaction from organized medicine that caused financial distress to the doctor for a long time to come.

One last thought on this subject of living, lasting proof. There are thousands of similar stories of victims of heart disease and circulatory problems . . . victims lucky enough to hear about chelation therapy and receive threatment. Unfortunately those numbers that have received treatment are very small compared to the large overall population of heart disease victims . . . some disabled permanently, others on life sustaining drugs and others just believing there are no answers to this killer problem.

Notice in the stories you have just read that patients usually remarked about feeling better after only a few treatments. I wondered why most all felt improved the same way I did, and were therefore encouraging themselves to continue their optional treatments. As I continued to read and gain more medical knowledge on circulatory problems, it finally dawned on me. Why did we all feel better in so short a time? The answers . . . you have already read about and there's more coming.

In simple terms, nutrient and oxygen carrying blood is getting into more areas of the body that have been shut-out from their life-giving benefits. Now metabolism is more complete, there's no shunting of enzyme activity, vitamin or mineral supplementation. The chemical plant is functioning better.

I also wondered about the role of the cardiolgist and heart surgeon in attending and treating my own heart problem as well as the thousands of other victims past, present and future. I realize now more than ever how lucky I am, and that I almost fell victim to their urging (for bypass surgery). Now what could I do to convince this multitude of coronary victims that there is truly a better and safer way . . . I am doing it now . . . Will you help?

NOTE: Some case histories were furnished courtesy of the National Health Federation of Monrovia, Calif., 91016. In their bulletin dated 2/80. Their publication is now called *Public Scrutiny*.

SUMMARY THOUGHT!

The weakness of human nature, here is personified by success stories of life saving importance that do not grow in emphasis and enthusiasm. but usually die in busy everyday living. We need a system here to propagate such successes. Do you have one?

Chapter Nine

UNFOUNDED OBJECTIONS

"He's a devout believer in witchcraft . . . called medical science."
. . . George Bernard Shaw

Let me first state a possible misunderstanding that may occur among some readers. Not every physician belongs to the American Medical Association, nor does he need to belong in order to practice medicine. The AMA membership is only representative of about 40% of all doctors. He can belong if he chooses, or some to affiliated County or State Medical Associations, or none. It does not harm his practice except if he belongs to such allied associations in some states or practices some non-approved AMA Therapy. Here pressure may be applied in various ways because of chelation therapy treatments or other therapy he may administer.

The AMA spells out EDTA for treatment of artheriosclerosis and related disorders as "useless because the effects are not lasting." Moreover, it considers the use of EDTA as "investigational." This was the discussion of the AMA council on new drugs in 1966. Yes, you read right . . . 1966. To my knowledge, no more recent appraisal has been officially made.

Before and during this time and still now EDTA is used under like conditions for the treatment of metallic poisoning (lead poisoning). Treatment is still performed and is still approved for this identical therapy as we are discussing for hardening of the arteries. Lead like calcium in the plaque (both minerals) as build-up, can be "cleaned out" by chelation therapy.

The March, 1977, issue of *Newsweek* contained an article about a chemical plant employee who ingested the largest amount of isotope Americanium 241 ever recorded. Harold McCloskey, age 64, said his life was saved by the treatment of the calcium salt of EDTA that is banned for treatment of hardening of the arteries. He is completely recovered, thanks to chelation therapy.

Surely these incidents do not make sense. Yes you can, but no you can't. There is contradiction by the FDA, but this means little to such a powerful government agency. They are pledged to enforcement of their guidelines.

The federal Government (FDA) backs these statements in spite of the fact that EDTA was at one time recognized as "possibly effective in occlusive disorders." Chelation was "wished away" when the quasi-recommendation was later withdrawn and in some states just legislated away. What has happened? Surely you can draw your own conclusions.

There are stories that would literally "turn your stomach" of harrassment to physicians performing this needed therapy. The AMA, FDA, local and state associations allied to the AMA, and related influential legal bodies, continually coerced and harrassed, from California to Florida. The shameful stories would fill a book larger than the Bible.

Dr. Morton Walker, in his excellent reporting thesis, "How to Reverse Hardening of the Arteries," tells of a patient of Dr. Harold W. Harper . . . Mrs. Ophelia Clementino. This is truly an emotional narration of an elderly woman, a victim of several strokes, who gradually became comotose from a series of added strokes and blood clots. This strong women hung in there; her throat muscles paralyzed, no urinary control, mindless, with feet swollen out of proportion. She lost weight and looked the picture of death.

The grown children of Mrs. Clementino, in their deep love, refused to believe the findings of the various doctors who had attended to her. They said there was nothing more they could do for her . . . "make her comfortable and she will slowly slip away."

Mrs. Clementino hung on despite nine strokes and finally her family was put in touch with Dr. H. Ray Evers of the Columbia General Hospital in Andulsia, Alabama. Upon hearing of the serious condition of the patient on the telephone, Dr. Evers thought a trip to his hospital would be too dangerous. He recommended they contact Dr. Harold W. Harper in California.

Dr. Harper called Mrs. Clementino as "so bad off she could have dropped dead at any moment." After an extensive examination, Dr. Harper warned the family of the mothers almost hopeless condition and of impending problems, but recommended they could try chelation therapy, since they were all so intent in their love for their mother. After long discussions, the family finally decided to go ahead with the chelation treatment since that hope was far more than the doctors at the hospital had given them.

To make matters worse, and after diligent preparation at St. Joseph's Hospital, the admittance of Mrs. Clementino, and the treaments having been instructed, rehearsed, and ready to start; the chairman for experimental medicine at the hospital refused to allow the treatment to start. After all sorts of arguing and threats, Mrs. Clementino had to be moved out of the hospital as Dr. Harper's pleadings were of no avail. It seemed that the hospital's excuse had to do with responsibility for a non-endorsed procedure and the condition of the patient.

The family searched and finally found an old run-down convalescent home to perform the treatments in. After much preparation by the family members, including cleaning and disinfecting the room, Mrs. Clementino was moved in. Dr. Harper had to start the infusions normally performed by a nurse and then had to instruct nurses on any possible emergency that could occur.

By the fifth treatment, her neurological responses had begun to return to her paralyzed right side. The process through succeeding treatments is really a heart-rendering story of gradual steady recovery. Her bowel movements had been controlled; she was eating; had control of her hands again; and finally shortly after was sitting on the side of the bed. Some time later, she was walking a little and finally later on was able to do what she wanted to do . . . "walk" out of the convalescent home. And finally still later to be able to walk into Dr. Harper's office for the first post-treatment visit. Mrs. Clementino received about 42 treatments spread over various intervals. (The entire emotional story is contained in Morton Walker's book.)

But that isn't the end of the story . . . by no means.

George W. Kell, an attorney of Modesco, California, represented Mrs. Clementino in her fight for payment under Medicare, parts A and B. At the Fair Hearing under Medicare she was told she could not collect under part B of the Medicare Act, after the carrier for Medicare, Occidental Life Insurance, turned down her request.

According to the line of thinking of the chief witness for Medicare, Dr. Soffer, Mrs. Clementino in so many words should have been allowed to die. This and the remarks of the doctors at the first hospital did not set well with the family and the attorney.

Attorney Kell disagreed and stated that had not chelation therapy been administered, the claimant would not have survived any more than a few days, and that chelation and EDTA was responsible for her recovery. Also that the witness, Dr. Soffer, along with his thinking, represented the feelings of the Administrator of St. Joseph's Hospital, which refused to permit personnel to administer life-saving treatment. The various parties representing the medical establishment condemned the patient to death because they did not believe in or have the knowledge of the treatment proposed; that Mrs. Clementino's former physicians and St. Joseph's Hospital had professional liability in the case.

While Mrs. Clementino lost the Medicare appeals. A later court decision in California stated, every doctor and hospital facility must explain *all* the proper alternatives. The court in *Cobb's vs. Grant* (8 CAL.3d, 229, 240; 104C.R. 505, 513) said every doctor owed the "duty and responsiblity of reasonable disclosure of available choices with respect to the proposed therapy and of the dangers inherently and patently involved in each," to his patients.

Said the Court, The doctor or hospital that fails to deliver the best product for the patient or withholds therapy offering less danger to the patient, which the doctor or the hospital has power to provide, may be guilty of malpractice. The court further held that a person of adult years of sound mind, or his responsible agent, has the right, in the exercise of control over his own mind and body, and to determine his own course of treatment. Ignorance of treatment is also tantamount to malpractice, the court ruled.

Consider the case of the pioneer in chelation, H. Ray Evers, M.D., a veritable martyr to the chelation cause. Dr. Evers was harrassed by the FDA, threatened with jail, revocation of his medical license, coevasive tactics, closing a hospital that caused his subsequent moves to other states. His medical skills and talents as a doctor for thirty-eight years were threatened and denied to his patients. The power of the government in coercion, harassment, legal talent backed by the law as interpreted, was finally won by Dr. Evers, little by little, on appeal after appeal. Dr. Evers was finally able to resume his practice again, a little wiser but poorer from expensive attorney and appeals costs.

The FDA's big guns then entered an anti-chelation attack on Dr. Evers. They seized the hospital inventory of EDTA. Dr. Evers countered with his usual civil suit in Federal Court. An injunction was granted Dr. Evers againts the FDA. Now the bureaucracy brought in the Internal Revenue Service. The IRS tried to impound his car until Dr. Evers resisted. So the IRS tried to indict him on a felony charge. Even with the help of the IRS, the FDA could not make the charges stick. The FDA lost the battle but won the war in causing substantial expense again.

It was here that the government influenced Medical Board of Louisiana stepped in and sought to inflict rules regarding hospital supervision. Finally, the examining board closed the hospital. Dr. Evers, after 26 months of legal battles and harassment, $142,000 in legal fees gone, remained without a license to practice medicine in Louisiana.

Dr. Evers moved to Montgomery, Alabama, and leased a 40-bed clinic where he offered patients from all over the United States, chelation therapy. The FDA attacked again with another lawsuit and on another angle of the law. Dr. Evers had 200 or more witnesses to testify for him, all former patients. The U.S. Judge ruled finally that the government or anyone else has no right to determine how a doctor should practice; that he was doing nothing wrong as a doctor; that he had the right to choose the method of treatment. No one could interfere with his rights to practice medicine. This ruling protected every physician in the United States, and still does.

There was still much harassment, and Dr. Evers finally decided it was best to get away from this official interference with his practice. He has since moved out of the United States and has opened a clinic and is practicing in the Bahamas.

The people in California were also affected by the restriction of chelation therapy. It is now permitted in that state after many off and on legal encounters with the California Medical Association. All legal encounters were fought tooth and nail by courageous physicians who practiced preventive medicine and administered chelation therapy. Of course, they had the help of thousands of satisfied patients in the court skirmishes. Possibly it was to much publicity over the miraclous help given to so many patients that encouraged harassment. Strict guidelines have been finally won on appeal and consistant proof of chelation therapy's merits is available to the public.

These dedicated physicians who had administered chelation therapy all these years had been stopped by various means of supression, conspiracy, threats to their state licensing, threats to loss of insurance coverage and many other tactics by the CMA.

It is interesting to note that California has more member Doctors in the American Academy of Medical Preventics than any other ten states of the United States. That AAMP was organized by these same pioneers to promote education and treatment of degenerative diseases, and to ensure public awareness of alternative methods of holistic medicine. This legal conspiracy to supress chelation therapy is stronger in California than anywhere else. I can only assume that the AMA has supported their allied association the CMA and their defensive and coersive efforts against chelation therapy more in California than anywhere else, this being the "root" of their overall opposition in the rest of the country.

The AMA has a new champion in their defense of any new therapy and new drugs coming on the health care scene. The angel . . . the Food and Drug Administration. They have their member physicians scattered throughout FDA bureaucratic empire.

Hardly ever does a new entry come upon us that the FDA cannot handle adequately with their strict 1962 guidelines passed into law by that Congress. So the AMA needs only to be behind the scene overseeing, possibly a little back door prodding, some innuendo, some occassional advice.

Basically the guidelines state there is need to prove efficacy and safety and to control testing with double-blind tests and controlled studies before approval of any therapy or new drug. The only valid criticism of EDTA chelation therapy is that very large, multivariant, double-blind controlled studies, at a cost of millions of dollars, have yet been conducted. Over the years various national institutions of health have consistantly refused to award any money for such research. Because the patent on EDTA has expired and no pharmaceutical company will invest in research. What results is a "Catch 22" situation in which funds for research will not be awarded because treatment is allegedly not effective, and in order to satisfy critics that the treatment is indeed effective such large scale studies must first be conducted.

Drug testing usually comprises litigation, the testing procedures for at least three years and several millions of dollars to the sponsoring company before the drug is even advertised and put up for initial sale. The result high drug prices.

My question is: Why can the AMA, without any official testing or procedure just start doing bypass surgery, maiming and losing some patients in the process, get away with this without any controls at all, no FDA sanction pro or con, and continue without opposition? Chelation therapy however already proven, with no lives lost remains unapproved. Draw your own conclusions.

Take, for instance, the FDA ruling with the controversial drug, GH3 or Gerovital H3. This is not a new drug. GH3 is a slight variation of a formulation in use for many years. The main part procaine, a deriative of novacaine, used for decades in the treatment of dentistry to heart disease arrhythmias. GH3 was discovered in Bucharest, Romania, and it is claimed to halt the aging process and keep people younger longer. The drug has been tested extensively all over the world by more than 500 laboratory studies conducted by leading physicians, scientists, and gerontologists (including in the U.S.). Nothing to my knowledge has been published on

GH3 by the Journal of the AMA. There is much evidence that it is useful as an antidepressant, makes cells reproduce longer, and increases muscular vigor.

Here is the information the FDA determined was necessary in order to prove to the FDA the merits of GH3 for the approval:

Patients with a depressive syndrome usually manifest depressed moods plus a significant number of associated symptoms. The FDA listed *15 symptoms* they consider for this depressed mood. The recommended *three phases* of testing consisted of:

(1) Patients already under psychiatric care, to determine safety and efficacy in the dosage prescribed. These patients would be withdrawn from all other drugs.

(2) Double blind studies in which GH3 would be tested against a placebo (harmless inert substance) under identical circumstances. The experiment would be devised so that the ampules would be identical in appearance; neither doctor nor patient would know what was being injected. In fact, no human being would know, because a third scientist working with a computer, independent of the testing group, would establish a code number for each ampule. The code would be sealed and broken only when the experiment was over. Only then would anyone know the results. Meanwhile, these patients would receive a battery of just about all the physical and mental tests known to medical science before, during, and after the experiment.

(3) The last test consists of GH3 being tested by 20 to 30 psychiatrists throughout the country, each working with 30 to 40 patients. This mushrooming action would ensure GH3 safety and confirm its efficacy on a relatively large scale, including the degree of allergic responses from these numbers.

The reason for phase (3) three mass testing is to find if a dangerous drug such as thalidomide which maimed hundreds of unborn children in a certian period of the mother's pregnancy, could be found. However, for every thalidomide, there are hundreds of potentially excellent drugs going unmarketed because of these too stringent laws passed in the wake of the thalidomide hysteria. All this is the opinion of many scientists and even some members of the FDA. Can you imagine the restrictions placed on a risky-close-to-death heart patient in a test procedure or doomed cancer patient?

This testing, as you can see, is too restrictive, too expensive, and too time-consuming. There must be some middle ground developed between safe and dangerous. Take penicillin, for instance; it could never pass the tests today. It is dangerous to a few, yet it has saved thousands of lives and opened the door for a new era in antibiotics in medicine. Aspirin too would not pass the present FDA tests as it causes internal bleeding and other problems taken in excess, and it still is not known why it works.

Right now the need is to save billions of dollars in Social Security payments for heart victims; Medicare payments of over two billion dollars for heart disease alone; to say nothing of the billions paid out by private insurance carriers . . . the result is staggering. And all of this money is ours, paid out needlessly, and chelation therapy approval is still withheld.

In chelation therapy the drug EDTA has already been approved for lead poisoning by the same method of administration. Yet the FDA has termed chelation therapy dangerous and says it has not been established in arteriosclerotic disease. This seems ridiculous and reeks of AMA influence of the FDA.

The need to change the FDA status on chelation therapy from "possibly effective" to "proven effective" will cost a group of some 200 dedicated AAMP doctor members close to 8 million dollars. What can we, the patients, do to help this situation? How can we help have chelation classified as preventive therapy for everyone? How can we convince the government that this therapy should be paid for by Medicare and that it is the cheapest way to prevention and the best bargain for the government? (See last two chapters)

This is the status of a preventive therapy that has saved thousands of lives and alleviated suffering for thousands more. Each year, heart disease increased from 6 to 9 percent more and still the AMA and the FDA ignore chelation therapy and condemns many doctors who use it. There's something wrong here in America . . . that must be revealed to Washington. This is the only place in the world with such health problems and so called protective laws. It's costing us billions of dollars and (and thousands of lives) that we can ill afford to pay with the pressures of inflation. We need your help, Dear Reader, for your voice to be heard, with others, now, when it counts the most.

The stories of medical and government harassment of doctors still goes on, and it will continue until *we the people* demand of our elected representative to bring this shameful situation to an end, and allow their health to be extended, their medical costs and taxes reduced, and their way of life improved.

It is time the medical establishment itself began looking for an even better treatment than chelation and spent their time in research rather than foster legal and coersive means to save their own selfish interest. It is time also for them to stop harassing doctors in their own profession.

Since the profit from chelation is comparatively low and the harrassment so high, I wondered why these dedicated men, members of the AAMP*, persisted in practicing chelation when there are other treatments and more profitable avenues to pursue. All I can say is they have a "compassionive feeling" for people, and are dedicated to their oath of healing the sick. Their prevention therapies are commendable and fruitful.

REFERENCES:

How to Prevent or Reverse Hardening of the Arteries, by Morton Walker, D.P.M.; '76 Press, P.O. Box 2686, Seal Beach, CA 90740.

GH3; Will it keep you young longer? by Herbery Bailey; Banton Books Inc., 666 Fifth Avenue, New York, NY 10019.

SUMMARY THOUGHT!

History shows its common practice . . . the power and might of money and influence in todays world bodes well of itself. But such power begets more power and unselfish deeds mount to a final reckoning and the undoing of the culprit.

*The American Academy of Medical Preventics is a non-profit organization and educational society for health care professionals interested in the prevention and/or treatment of chronic degenerative diseases. The Academy's goals are to improve the skills, knowledge, and diagnostic procedures, and to ensure the public awareness of alternative holistic methods of prevention and treatment.

Chapter Ten
NOW I BELIEVE IN NUTRITION

"The number of years we live is not nearly as important (life span) if they are miserable years."

. . . Richard Passwater, Ph.D.

Nutrition is a field that out of self defense and my condition I was told I needed to learn. I received reliable information by association with preventive physicians and at their suggestions regarding recommended books.

Nutrition is a field filled with many theories and few facts; consequently, it is easy for exploiters of doubt to peddle "magic potions" and fad diets. There are no standards or certification required to become expert(?) in this quickly changing field. This is one reason why I never became too interested in vitamins and supplements in the past.

We now know of chelation therapy, and the help provided to help relieve hardening of the arteries and other related diseases, to give new life to cells and repair any tissue damage, to improve circulation, to receive life-giving oxygen to the *entire body*. Now we need to *feed* the entire body back to continueng health, an important part of holistic medicine. If we don't the chelation is wasted.

It was explained to me by my physician that chelation therapy was only a part of the overall treatment on my way back to complete recovery. Nutrition plays the metabolic part of the treatment. That prevention of the recurrence of a heart attack was just as important. That vitality and energy taken away in ever-increasing increments since the passage of our 20th year of life was equally important to gain back. That I can live a full enjoyable life into the future. In other words, I cannot go from McDonald's to Mommas too quickly.

As I read and continued the holistic approach I became a "believer." I want you to become a believer also so that you, too, can become a like example of good health and vitality. Since nutrition is a technical subject, I do not intend to involve readers in an easily misunderstood subject. So we will stick to plain, and I hope easy reading facts I have learned from the experts.

Nutritionists can be in any of four categories: M.D.'s ' Ph.D's; dieticians; and "others." Doctors with a degree in nutrition are hard to find, which no doubt is why so many people looking for help and knowledge have changed to "others." Lately a few medical schools and some graduate schools have been graduating doctors with a degree in nutrition. You have to look a long time to find someone who hangs out a shingle declaring expertise in nutrition. I have found you can waste money & time and many recommendations are not too beneficial, many of these "experts" put on a good show and sell product. All the professional medical groups mentioned in chapter one qualify. These physicians and scientists make nutrition the heart of their practice just as the conventional physician prescribes drugs.

But heart disease is a product of modern lifestyles; of the lack of proper nutrition. Many believe a change of lifestyles back to the "good old days" is all that is required to prevent their heart problem. This would help, but the food we eat and the environment of today is not like the "good old days."

Dr. Roger Williams, the doctors recognized authority and pioneer in nutrition has had many thoughts on the subject.

He has said that the brain is the "hot spot" of chemical activity. An adult brain weighing only three or four percent of our body weight is where chemical burning takes place. This could be 25% of the body's total weight. Fuel needs to be supplied for this task every minute of the day as brain cells need to be maintained to carry on the active burning.

The Doctor maintains that brain cells do not get proper nutrition, that they limp along with what ever nutrition they can get. To make matters worse it is estimated that 1000 cells die off in an adult every hour. If these cells are not replaced they die off because of poor nutrition. Brain cells die off more rapidly than other cells.

For example alcohol consumption is poor nutrition. The brains of an alcoholic after death reveal the useless dissection by medical students resulting in a structureless mush. Likewise when we combine the "refined" materials of plants an animals (sugar, starch and fats) we get mostly fuel and little building blocks of nutrition to maintain our body organs.

Dr. Williams has stated we must ask ourselves how to get into our bodies and internal environment the best assortment of raw materials possible, if our living cells are to subsist.

Many Americans suffer each year from diseases that nutrition could prevent. America is malnurished. Great numbers of foods are mislabeled and designed to protect their previous evaluations that are outdated. This includes evaluation the FDA, the USDA, various doctors advice. TV advertising, and food manufacturers. These are the people who say if you meet USDA recommended daily requirements (RDA) or minimum daily requirements (MDA) you are being fortified adequately. It's like looking at a new car sticker and believing the city and country miles per gallon that is stated; both are inaccurate.

Something happened to me since I began chelation therapy treatments. While many may think it unimportant . . . I think it is significant and important enought to mention here, possibly proof that something is right in these chelation treatments and with nutrition.

For probably 25 years I have had a large mole on my left temple located just above and behind the eye and near where the hairline starts. I always thought of having it removed as its top looked like a black wart on dead skin lying on a big pimple. It made me look old, like age spots I see so often

A few weeks ago I noticed the dead skin part, the top, become partially detached; so I put some medication on it so it would heal without causing a problem. Finally a few days later, washing it caused it to come off, but there was no bleeding. A few days later the pimple part was gone also . . . all gone completely after 25 years . . . why?

The second thing happened while I am having chelation treatments, and afterwards for several hours. I have had a chronic prostate problem for about 20 years. It has never caused any more than the usual fine stream, frequent urination in two stages and a long drip afterwards. During the chelation and for about that day, the stream increases to possibly three times it usual size (to me it looks like the dam just broke). Why? I don't know. I do know that I am passing some metal taken out by the treatment; zinc and manganese is recommended to help prostate problems.

The third happening . . . I am now able to push the lawn mower, dig in the yard, and bend and stoop over for long periods of time. Before my heart attack I was on a dilating drug because I got dizzy spells when I stooped over. My doctor claimed the artery going up my neck to my head was partially blocked, and he proved it. That artery must be clear now as I don't have any dizzy spells anymore. There must be a relationship between chelation and nutrition; this I believe.

In a 1971 report of the United States Department of Agriculture, Dr. Weir estimated that if all American diets were improved to government level recommended daily allowances (RDA), there would be dramatic improvements in at least 19 major health problems and one-half million lives saved yearly. Among the benefits are the following estimates:

• 25% reducation in heart disease incidence and death; 300,000 lives saved.

• 20% reduction in cancer incidence and death; 150,000 lives saved.

• 10,000,000 more elderly without impairment.

• 14% to 20% fewer days lost per person from work alone, due to respiratory infections.

• Slashed arthritis incidence, diabetes, and infant mortality reduced by half.

• 3,000,000 fewer children born without birth defects.

That forecast is not exaggerated when you figure out what supernutrition can do for you. RDA values fluctuate, with 55 major changes made in the last 15 years, and are suspect . . . based on conflict of interest and the self-serving views of certain food industry people. At any rate the government minimums really mean many Americans are not getting even minimum nutrition requirements.

"In our youth our cell replacement exceeds the rate of cell deaths. Our young bodies compensate for lack of nutrients as they grow. As youths reach teen age, Americans are building future misery for themselves from the food they eat. These bad habits will show up 20 to 30 years later," says Richard Passwater. This already has been proven.

Nature's rule is that life shall feed upon life. But there are today, spoiling and detrimental effects on food nutrients by cooking, transportation, soil depletion, storage, exposure to light and heat, etc.

The need to prepare foods properly becomes more important. For instance:

- Don't fry foods; it destroys protein.
- Use very little water in cooking. Add the cooked water back to the meal with soluble vitamins.
- If possible, eat raw foods more.
- Avoid storage. Buy smaller quantities.
- Keep food as cold as possible in storage.

Natural foods are great . . . since all foods originally come from living plants and animals. The health of ancient people, their strength and size attest to this. This is the kind of food which Mother Nature designed for the human body. We should eat natural foods as much as possible.

I have found Granola bars a good snack food to eat. Natural cereal such as "proteinola" is my most delicious discovery. I mix fresh fruit or raisins with it. It is also very filling. My stomach is satisfied more easily. This is something I found that other cereals lacked. Likewise toasted soybeans sure tops peanuts for food and for health.

Almost every name-brand cereal contains an alarming amount of sugar; up to 52 percent in Kellogg's Apple Jacks, and many other brands have just as much.

Sugar depletes the body's stores of certain vitamins and minerals vital to normal function; causes hypoglycemia (low blood sugar); and, among other things, is believed to be a cause of children becoming hyperactive.

Sugar and its effects are discussed in the chapter entitled, "The Bad White Stuff."

The cereals found in health food stores use only natural sweeteners (fructose) found in dates and raisins or sometimes honey. They are high in fiber, which provides important bulk that helps your digestive system regulate itself. They have no artificial colors or flavors, are low in sodium, and very filling without the empty calories.

The key words in nutrition are "enzyme" and "antioxidant". Antioxidant is a substance that prevents oxidation (reaction with oxygen) by combining with the oxygen. Enzymes are the chemical backbone of metabolism. Nothing happens in the metabolic or internal biochemical arena without enzymes. Chemical reactions can occur almost immediately in the body by the action of enzymes. One area of activity is the digestive tract where enzymes play an intergral part in the conversion of foods into utilizable nutrients. The other area of activity is internal, or within the cellular structure. All biochemical and metbolic reactions need enzymes **for activation.** Enzyme laden foods strengthen both enzyme systems. *Heat destroys enzymes.* This again means that raw foods are best. Cooked foods kill enzyme activation so you need an abundance of enzymes to be taken orally for good nutrition, if you eat too many very hot cooked foods.

Critical in avoiding heart disease are the B-Complex vitamins. These form co-enzymes that metabolize the fat and sugar in our diet. B6 is also part of the co-enzyme that helps form lecithin, which is like a detergent and keeps cholesterol and fats soluble in the blood. The more B12 you eat the better, particularly if you are on a vegetarian diet.

The growing interest in Vitamin E in most diets, and Vitamin C (both are more than just ordinary vitamins) are important enought to discuss in detail in a later chapter.

Vitamin and mineral supplements help the following:

- Reduce the need for tranquilizers.
- Correct enzyme deficiency.
- The common cold via Vitamin C.
- Water pollution.
- Iron lost in menapause.
- Skin cancer.
- Using the "pill."
- Hypoglycemia and sugar.
- Dieting needs vitamins.
- Heart disease.
- Deactivate cancer-causing chemicals.
- Sexual pleasure increased.
- Protects cell membranes against cancer-causing chemicals.
- Stay young longer.

Selenium—according to Passwater is a protector, this mineral element protects our cells from cancer, heart problems and premature old age. Found in only certain areas of the country—the selenium should be taken in tablet form regularly. Current research should reveal strong evidence on the merits of this needed mineral.

The name of the game is that a healthy cell is not a sick cell. Sick cells die unless they receive an extra supply of nutrients known to help, including oxygen.

Certain bad habits are inconsistent with your search for health. You cannot build a castle with one hand and expect to tear it down with the other. Alcohol, for instance, has proven destructive to brain cells as well as liver cells, both vital to good health.

Smoking . . . you know all the evidence. It is carcinogenic and destroys Vitamin C. Smoking creates more work for the liver to detoxify the toxic products of cigarette smoke.

The overconsumption of coffee and tea that contains habit-forming drugs can harm the central nervous system. I drink one cup of coffee each morning. That's it.

Calcium is important in reducing irritability of nerves and muscles. Get's rid of "charlie horses." Calcium helps utilize the balance of sodium, magnesium, phosphorous and potassium, as well as Vitamin D. They all work together helping to metabolize calcium.

Calcium is used by the heart in muscle contraction that provides the heartbeat, and magnesium repels the calcium to reverse contraction to allow the heart to relax. Hardness in water is mainly calcium and magnesium. (See chapter on water)

Potassium is very important. It is the intercellular electrolyte of as great importance as sodium is for extracellular fluid. Lacking potassium causes weakness of the nerves supplying the heart muscle, which in turn sends blood into the circulatory system.

Cane sugar and processed carbohydrates demand B-Complex vitamins in order to be processed through the metabolic biochemical channels within the body. When the B vitamins are stolen from other areas of metabolism or chemical activity, they create deficiencies in the metabolic areas and problems can result. One area affected is the nervous system. In relation to the heart, this means that nerve control of the rate of rhythm of the heart can be altered; and the development of cardiac arrythmias or abnormal pulsations occur.

Synthetic fats and chemicals in the diet and environment are taken into the body one way or another. These substances are **not foods;** they contain no micronutrients. Therefore **they must steal** the essential vitamins, minerals, and enzymes from other areas of metabolism in order to be metabolized out of the body. So these fats are nutritional deficiencies that are taken into the body in increasing numbers.

The combination of hardened arteries that cause a reduction in blood flow when coupled with any of the above factors will develop and increase angina pain. (Better read again)

The over-consumption of fats, mostly saturated fats, as well as sugar, salt, cholesterol, and alcohol have definite relationships to six of the ten leading causes of death; heart disease, cancer, cerebrovascular disease, diabetes, artheriosclerosis, and cirrohis of the liver. Dietary trends, too, may be leading to malnutrition through undernourishment because fats and refined sugars are very low in vitamins and minerals.

What to do? Here are some suggestions:

(1) Eat your foods as near natural form as possible. About 60 percent of your food supply is processed; that is, puffed up, stripped down, emulsified, thickened, and/or dosed with chemicals. Processed foods are high in sugar, salt, fat, and additives. Catsup is 26 percent sugar by weight.

(2) Use lemon juice spices and herbs as flavorings instead of salting your food. Don't use foods with visible salt such as pretzels, potato chips and crackers.

(3) Read the ingredient label on all food products; the first ingredients are the prominent ones in order down the list. Make label reading a habit at the table.

(4) Try to bake your own bread and cakes (without using cake mixes). Most commercially-made baked goods and some dried soups contain powdered eggs which are even higher in fats & cholesteral than regular eggs.

(5) Use frozen vegetables when fresh vegetables are not available. The canned versions are very high in salt.

(6) Avoid products with either **coconut oil** or **palm oil,** such as coffee lighteners. They are both vegetable oils

and are high in saturated fats and used in most food processing. The word hydrogenated fats spell problems.

(7) Decrease your meat consumption; beef, pork and lamb are high in fat. Eat light fresh fish (dark fish is higher in fat), poultry, and vegetable proteins. Incomplete protein such as beans and rice become complete when eaten together.

THE TEN WORST FOODS . . . AND BRIEF REASONS

SUGAR	Empty calories; poor after-effects.
RED MEAT	Fat; additives from cattle feed.
WHITE BREAD	Additives are cancer causing; preservatives are nutrient-deficient non-foods.
ALCOHOL	Empty calories; nutrition damage; bad diet.
COW'S MILK	Allergy-causing; salt; fat sugar; protein; lactose.
LUNCH MEAT	Nitrites cancer-causing; salt; not grown but manufactured.
FRIED FOOD	Bad fat; little nutrients; some vitamins but kills enzymes.
CAFFEINE	Heart problem; addiction; an upper (stimulant); hypertension and jangled nerves; vitamin antagonist; like nicotine; empty calories; bad after-effects.
DIET SOFT DRINKS	No nutrient value; not a thirst-quencher.
BREAKFAST CERALS	Additives; heat kills vitamins and enzymes; a dead food; the life force natural part is gone even though they put back vitamins.

Here are my own daily intake nutritional supplements I take religiously. They are listed as morning and evening doses although they comprise twice a day intake recommended for my personal use. Yours could vary in many ways depending on evaluations by your physician.

Morning Intake	Afternoon / Evening Intake
1 400 IU vitamin E	1 400 IU Vitamin E
1 500 mg vitamin C	1 500 mg Vitamin C
1 50 mcg selenium	1 45 mg chelated zinc
1 45 mg chelated zinc	1 45 mg magnesium
1 lecithin 20 minims	1 45 mg potassium
1 B Complex 50 mg each	1 B Complex 50

This B Complex vitamin has either 50 mg or 50 mcg of: Folic acid niacamide B 12, B6, & B1 pantothenic acid inositol and biotin.

I eat little or no breakfast or lunch. Because in addition I take Spirulina Tablets as a supplement and appetite supressant. Fifteen minutes before breakfast I take 3 500Mg Spirulina and 1, Spirulina Green Gold which has an added 500 mg of bee pollen, ginseng powder and papya enzyme, plus 500 mg of Spirulina. I take the same 4 tablets before dinner to help supress desire for food and for nutritional input. Spirulina is a blue green microalgae vegetable plankton containing the richest source of metabolic pigments, natural proteins (70%) and carotene (pro vitamin A). Six ½ gram tablets also provide 135 mg of DNA and RNA, 78mg of linoleic acid, 30-45 mg of chlorophyll, 25-50 mg of phycocyanin, 17, mcg of B6, 0.57 IU of Vitamin E and 1 MCG of selenium. Spirulina is grown naturally, is 95 percent digestable and appears to be coming on strong as a universal natural grown food with many benefits to health and weight control, naturally.

A QUICK CHECK LIST . . .

DESIRABLE FOODS

All garden vegetables, fresh and frozen preferred
Veal, lamb, beef, vension (all limited) fish and chicken
Trimmed steaks and chops broiled or stewed
Buttermilk, yogurt, cottage cheese, sourkraut
Fruits, fruit juices and fresh vegetable juices
Wheat bran, rice bran, oatmeal, wheat germ, wheat germ, Soy beans, sunflower seeds.

UNDESIRABLE FOODS

All sugar products, cola and soda drinks
Alcohol, coffee, tea, coca and low calorie drinks
Pie, cakes, crackers, puddings, candy

Hamburger, franks, meat loaf, sausage, chili, lunch meats, bacon, processed meats
Processed foods with sugar
White bread, white buns, biscuits, rools, spaghetti, macaroni pie crusts, doughnuts

There is no question that the media backed by the manufacturer has turned cereals into a nutritional hype. They tell you that you can get 100 percent of RDA from a breakfast cereal, they imply that you don't have to think about your diet for the rest of the day. That is brainwashing and absurd.

Readers may be puzzled by the use of words like Orthmolecular. This was coined by Dr. Linus Pauling, world renowned nutritionist. It means having the right molecules in the body in the right amounts. Megavitamin therapy is simply correcting the body's chemistry with extra large doses of food supplements. Preventive medicine fills both of these requirements as does holistic medicine. In all these various names there is only one basic difference from conventional medicine; they substitute in most cases food supplements for drugs. These modern medical practicioners rely on nature's way of correcting illness rather than changing the body chemistry with drugs.

And of course the powerful AMA opposes anyone who practices anything against their usual drugs and symptom theory. I speak with experience when I say this modern approach to treatment far excels anything that conventional medicine has come up with so far. We keep winning converts daily.

One last thought I read from the nutrition experts. There is a "grey zone" of only possible or non-proven results. Beware of the nutrition charlatans who could fill you with vitamins you may or may not need or who make tests that could be of questional value. There are store front experts where you are zipped through a procedure without a through work-up and proper relative testing. They will be promoting quick cures and many sophisticated tests that could spell trouble. So called nutritional experts (?) have typically had the loudest voices with the least educational research techniques. No wonder there is confusion that typifies the present nutrition business.

Chapter Eleven

PREVENTION . . . THE WAY OF LIFE

"The most effective water power in the world . . . woman's tears."
. . . Wilson Mizner

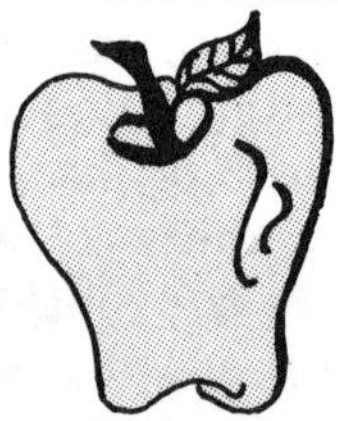

A very wise and talented old man once said, "The doctor of the future will give no medicine, but will interest his patients in the care of the human frame, in diet, and in the cause and prevention of disease."

–Thomas A. Edison

The modern approach to medical problems is being practiced today and becoming more popular as medical care costs increase. It is holistic medicine or preventive medicine depending on which physician who practices it wishes to call it. Holistic means treating both the mind and spirit as well as the whole body. Many physicians who practice Prevention are pioneers in this unhearlded segment of the medical profession. They have however, broken away from the AMA because of their true belief in curing the disease rather than treating the symptoms contineously. They also believe in the Hypocratic oath they took upon being awarded their degree as medical doctor.

Their approach to medicine is not only novel by today's standards, but proven most successful in the maintenance of continued good health. They also believe in and administer the controversial but highly effective chelation therapy with which this writer has had so much success.

In the therapeutic program I received, it was most satisfying to know that I was being treated, and most likely cured, of a lingering problem of hardening of the arteries, as well as (I hope) healing around a heart infarction, and unclogging the arteries that cause the angina pain.

The testing procedures were unusual but ultra-modern, some of which I had never heard of before. For instance, a computerized dietary analysis; a hair analysis that is returned in computer form; several different blood tests; a complete physical examination; and many other interesting tests that are optional, all this before anything in the way of therapy was attempted.

The hair analysis tells how, through diet, you can decrease your tendency toward blood vessel disease. Research has shown that hair more closely reflects the minerals in the body which are accumulating, than does the blood or urine, particularly in cases of toxic metal exposure. The analysis provides a readout of minerals in your body and indicates those in which it is deficient. Often the hair will show toxicity when the blood or urine tests will not. By adding the metals you are deficient in, you increase your overall level of health and nutrition. The second and equally important reason for this analysis is that chelation therapy tends not only to remove toxic minerals such as calcium, mercury and cadmium, but it also removes needed metals such as copper, zinc, magnesium and iron. Fortunately these needed trace elements are easily replaced.

Here are some highlights to this new and modern approach to hair analysis. A method also called Plasma Emission Spectroscopy, that should make hair analysis cost effective for everyone. The problem could be in the accuracy in various licensed labs who are supposed to operate under rigorous quality control.

This method, it is predicted, in time will take its place along with blood and uring analysis now widely accepted. Hair analysis offers hope that biochemical imbalances can be detected *"before"* they develope into diseases. To control our chemical factory from over producing or under-affecting body metabolism. There are four major areas where hair analysis can be extremely helpful:

1. Identification of long term excessive exposure to potentially toxic metals i.e. lead, cadmium, mercury, arsenic, nickel, aluminum from water, food and air. Some sources of lead exposure which most of us find hard to escape include tap water, canned foods, peeling paint, house dust, street

dirt, auto exhaust, leaded gasoline and hair dressings that prevent or reverse gray hair.

It has been used in tests for criminal detection correction from various convictions. Also to detect impaired student performance in the classroom.

2. Hair analysis is a useful screening test for the early identification of malabsorption and/or impaired digestion. This should allay the myths we see and hear on TV that all stomach upset is blamed on excess acidity.

3. Zinc/copper ratio. The recent headlines we have seen indict dietary cholesterol and fat as a cause of coronary artery disease in otherwise healthy persons. This zinc/copper ratio is an important indicator of development of artery disease and the indictment is erronious. Recent discoveries show that our bodies produce cholesterol each day in levels equal to 8 to 10 eggs. Our liver must function to break down this large amount down. This breakdown requires help from minerals such as copper. Hair analysis indicates the ratio of copper to other minerals which may be frequently antagonistic to chelation therapy. Nutritionists speak of zinc/copper ratio, just the proper amounts of any metal but not too much of any metal. Poisoning could happen in prolonged use of zinc or any metal. The zinc/copper ratio is a better predictor of potential heart disease or acclusive artery disease than any other commonly recognized risk factors such as serum cholesterol, blood pressure etc.

4. Calcium/mangesium. Our westernized diets have developed major health problems, among them gradual loss of calcium from bones and teeth, leading to serious demineralization of our skeleton, called osteoporosis, common to people over 50, mostly women. After a change of life many women lose their height as their bones settle down with a loss of strength. Fractures are prevelent as is loss of teeth. Hair analysis appears very promising as a most sensitive test to reveal those who are in a negative calcium balance at an earlier age.

NOTE: For a complete report on hair analysis from a scientific paper see the back pages.

Many patients ready to under-go chelation therapy believe that all they have to do is go in the clinic and receive treatment because they already know quite a bit about their disease, having been through many trying medical experiences already, some to the point of near death. They have already received positive diagnosis and have even been educated somewhat by these experiences. This all may be true, except for the fact that the doctor now must base his treatments on what he learns from his own tests.

Some question the taking of so many pills that are needed because they have never been exposed to supplements before, something new has been added. We could have a mineral deficiency as we have learned and we are reminded that the farmer must add trace minerals back into the soil so the soil is not deficient in them.

Vitamin/mineral programs are designed for each patient indivdiually, as part of the prevention program. These supplements are usually obtained in a drug or health food store and it is an important part of the overall program.

The final reason is the discrepancy between modern nutritionists' thinking about our diet and what the Federal Government (USDA) thinks with their recommended daily requirements (RDA) and ever changing standards. Such standards have been challenged since their inception and opinions abound at every official change. Nutritionists think the standards are too low.

BLOOD TESTS. These tests usually indicate actual organ disease, and it is done on initial evaluation with an extensive inventory of blood tests. This is to insure that your liver and kidneys are able to handle the therapy. In addition, the function of the blood tests is to access factors that predispose you to blood vessel disease, mainly diabetes and blood-fat elevations. As you progress these are monitored periodically, and further tests performed.

PLETHYMOGRAPHY is a safe technique for measuring externally the blood flow through the arm, leg, head and neck vessels. It measures the elasticity of the vessels and indicates the rate and extent to which they expand. The rate of expansion and the elasticity or recoil of the arteries is important. This is assessed on the initial evaluation and usually between the 20th and 30th treatment. This technique is a determining factor in the progress of the therapy as comparisons of the readings are made. It is non-invasive and similiar to an electrocardiogram.

ELECTROCARDIOGRAPHY (EKG) is evaluated in three stages, mostly for the patients own benefit after the first. The preliminary EKG is the resting one that serves to tell if the heart is significantly diseased or if there are any pecularities in the rate of rhythm. Later the optional tests are for heart functions under stress and exercise.

It is possible to observe the back of the eye and the blood vessels there. This is accomplished by various methods to obtain clear observable indications if disease is present and to what degree. Heart disease often show up first in the eyes. So not only is the eye "the mirror of our soul; the eye is the mirror of our physiology. Retinal photography actually shows disease related changes and is not used by all physicians, other than opthomologists.

HOD DIAGNOSTIC TEST reveals nervous system functional disturbances that have a bearing on general health and well being.

DROPPLER TEST. An ultrasonic device to evaluate local blood flow alterations. This test obviates invasive methods such as Catheteration.

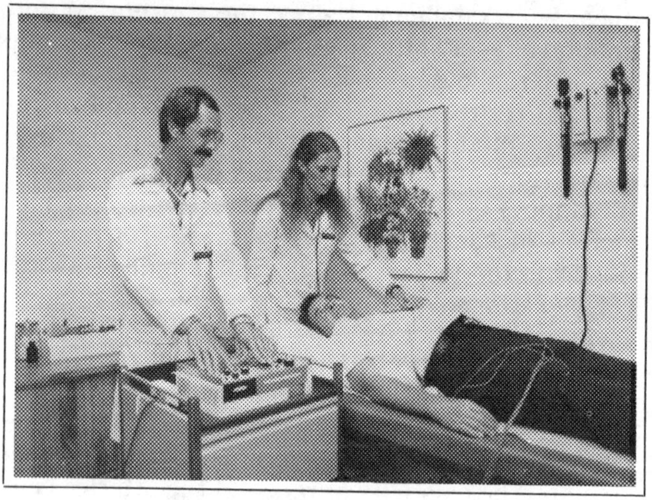

High density lipoproteins (HDL) have a protective or dissolving effect on the plaque in the arteries. It is necessary to evaluate the ratio of cholesterol to HDL to determine risk factors involved. Here the goal is to lower cholesterol and raise HDL level, dietarily and with vitamins, minerals and exercise. Your progress is monitored periodically to determine blood sugar, cholesterol, HDL, and another blood fat called trigIicerides.

In additon to the above there are glucose tolerance tests to evaluate sugar and energy metabolism that is necessary to provide power to drive all bodily functions, physically and mentally.

There is tubeless Heidleberg Gastrogram to evaluate stomach acid content to detect a degree of digestive capability needed for proper digestion and assimilation of food.

Where do we start seeking answers to disease? Where do we place the basic problem? We start right in our own bodies where our way of living has changed. Our chemical factory is forced into new reactions that upset the proper functioning of various organs. One part of the system is affected which in turn affects other parts. Ignorance and neglect play a part in this process but because of our body's ability to fight back with self help, we learn little from this process. The bulk of illness today arises from gradual and long-standing, but slow insidious breakdown in the bodies structure and function. Thus, repeated daily minute and multiple micro-insults damage bodily (cellular) function and

EFFECT OF RISK FACTORS ON INCIDENCE OF CORONARY EVENTS AND SUDDEN DEATH

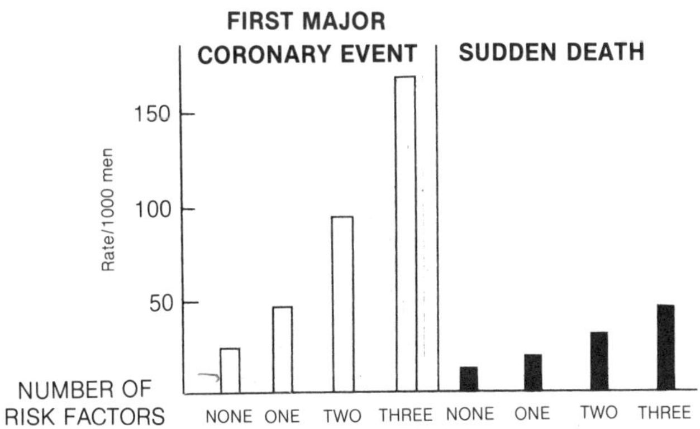

Relationship between the number of major risk factors (smoking, hypertension, and hypercholesterolemia) and the incidence of a first major coronary event and sudden death.

thereby produce metabolic alterations that result from, as well as cause, chemical imbalance, or call it malnutrition.

Many such bodily changes cause us to have a universal common denominator in the form of vascular degeneration. This obstruction interferes with the life preserving channels

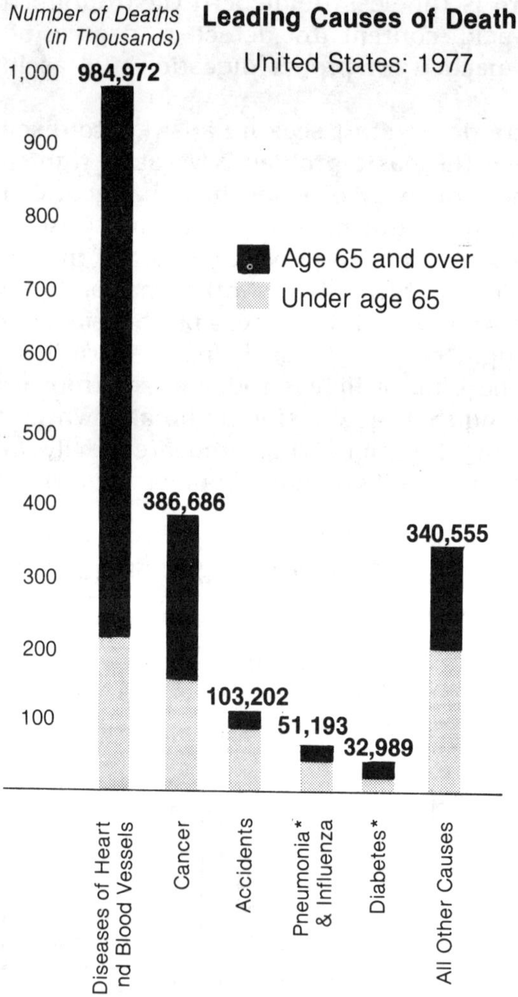

Source: National Center for Health Statistics,
U.S. Public Health Service, DHEW

*Deaths from suicide, certain causes of mortality in early infancy, cirrhosis of the liver, and homicide exceed those from pneumonia and influenza, and diabetes for persons under the age 65.

for our blood. The result is a gradual reduced blood supply and with it decreased nutrition to the various parts of the body. With it oxygen is reduced, nurishment to tissue is reduced and at the same time a build-up occurs of toxic waste products which further interferes with normal function.

A reduction in circulation results from a gradual accumulation of abnormal fat and mineral deposits on the lining and in the walls of the hollow pipe-like blood vessels. They start to take place in infancy and accumulate slowly year after year according to lifestyle. Then later this damage builds up to a point of breakdown in one or more parts of the body. This breakdown produces symptoms and signs with loss of physical activity and performance according to the importance and type of the cells involved.

Many people think it is old age setting in because we don't see it in children. Well, we do see it and there are cases of obstructions in children and even death from the problem as we will see later. We lose sight of the causes and facts because the changes are so gradual in most instances. Then there is Mother Nature's built-in tolerances that protect us to later years. This "masking" of our true condition, the eventual crisis resulting in various degenerative diseases, usually fail to occur until loss of nearly 90 percent of blood flow causes sypmtoms and disability, causing one to suddenly realize they are not well.

At this point we have been talking about a class of disease, a degenerative disease that indicates a breakdown in the normal regenerative repair and maintenance processes which normally preserves and promotes our health. We have tissues, organs and glands showing signs of wearing out.

There are other degenerative diseases that are reduced in function but less dramatic and relatively less life-threatening; diabetes, arthritis, parkinsonism to mention a few. All have one thing in common—reduced function of the involved diseased tissue, as a result of poor blood supply, which is a consequence of increased deposition of abnormal build-up of plaque in the blood vessel walls.

Hypertension or high blood pressure starts many of our illnesses. Many medical questionnaires seek answers that can help a diagnosis. "Ever had hypertension?" Now have hypertension? "no longer have hypertension? and "never had hypertension? They take in seven demographic characteristics of age, sex, family income, education, race, region of the country and place of residence. All these needed answers indicate if the person has had medical treatment that was successfully treated or not, and persons who were

High Blood Pressure More Than Triples the Risks of Heart Failure and Stroke.

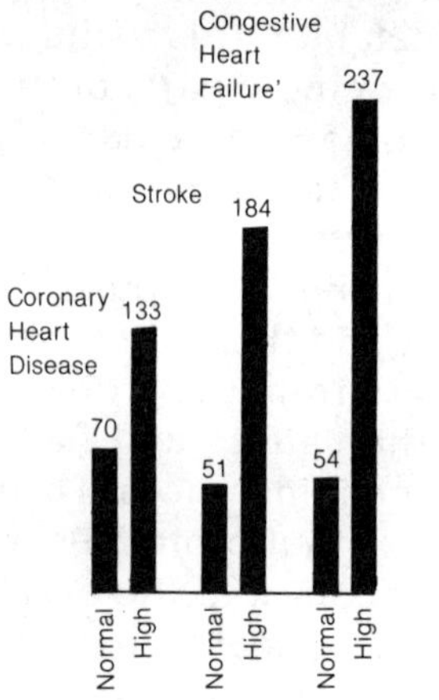

Number of Patients with Normal and High Blood Pressure

Deaths due to Cardiovascular Diseases by Major Type of Disorder United States: 1977

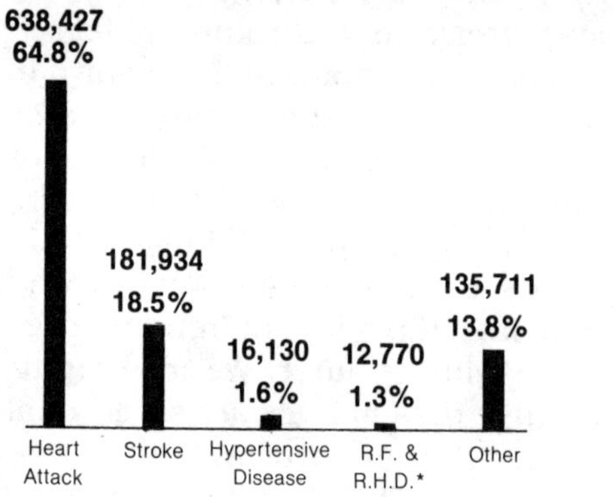

*Rheumatic Fever and Rheumatic Heart Disease
Source: National Center for Health Statistics, USPHS, DHEW

told they had hypertension, etc. All these statistics indicate the seriousness of hypertension and more importantly, its later effect on many developing diseases. So we look for the "tell tale signs."

To find these "tell tale" signs we must look to ourselves and our habits and lifestyles. In a later prevention chapter we will find some answers to our overall health problems.

NOTE: Not all the tests just mentioned are needed by every patient. This is an overview of most all the available tests. Your physician determines the tests that are needed, from his initial evaluations.

Chapter Twelve

WHO NEEDS BYPASS SURGERY?

"Culture is what your butcher would have, if he were a surgeon."
. . . Mary Pettibone Poole

Coronary bypass surgery may be the most momentous innovation in modern medicine. Approximately 100,000 bypass operations a year are performed in more than 500 hospitals, about 800 at the University of Alabama Hospital alone, at about $20,000 average cost per patient. That's over three billion dollars each year spent on this surgery alone. By 1986, if this enthusaism in the medical industry continues, it will be a $100 billion industry.

The operation was developed about 1964 to treat the largest cause, the #1 killer in the United States, coronary heart disease. The procedure involves bypassing the occluded or blocked portion of the **three** major arteries feeding into the heart, with vein grafts taken from the patients leg. There were great hopes and enthusism ran high when the procedure was introduced, as it relieved angina or chest pains and allowed the patient more activity, prevented frequent attacks and could prolong life.

Newspapers, magazines and television have dramatized the miraculous benefits of the new surgery. The intense and anxiety-provoking pain of the disease makes the heart patient eager to try anything that promises relief.

Fred and Bernie are brothers; Fred is 52 and Bernie is 56. Their father died of a heart attack when Bernie's age. Both Bernie and Fred have coronary artery disease. It is painful and at time incapacitating.

Bernie recently underwent open-heart surgery. He chose to have the operation "because the quality of life was important to me; I didn't want to spend the rest of my days not being able to be active and do all the things I like to do".

His brother, Fred, says, "There's no way they're going to get me on that table and saw me down the middle like a chicken. No way. Nothing I've read or heard has convinced me that surgery will do any good anyway. I'll take my chances."

These brothers with opposing views are indicative of the growing controversy over bypass surgery. This concern is high because conventional medicine and the media do not talk alternatives and too many victims never heard of chelation therapy. Actually, there are many more questions than there are positive answers.

A patient who has had a successful bypass operation must have faith and lives in hope that the operation he had will prolong his life. Unfortunately he does not know. Views of successes and failures are biased. Long term follow-up cannot be counted as valid proof (it has been expounded somewhat) of success because of the varied lifestyles pursued by the bypass patients. Do they change or continue on the same debilitating course that cause the problem? But the main first reaction by patients is that they are now free of pain, and they are able to exercise and start life all over again.

"The disease is a little strange," says Dr. Horace MacVaugh, chief of the Division of Throatic and Cardiovascular surgery at Lankenau Hospital, Philadelphia. He says artery disease affects people differently in areas of the body at different rates. **Many physicians agree there is evidence that almost everyone has it.** They mention autopsies of young men killed in Korea of about 19 and 21 years of age where remarkable advanced coronary lesions in many of them were found. More than 90 percent of these soliders had evidence of the disease, not as yet serious, but the evidence showed build up in most all of them.

A study by Dr. George Berenson, who directed a Louisiana State University project in Bogalusa, Louisiana, even found two-year-old children with cholesterol levels as high as those of young adults. Cholesterol levels are thought by many doctors to be related to coronary artery disease.

In any case, some people go through life showing no signs of artery disease. Other exhibit symptoms ranging from leg pain (caludication) after walking short distances, to various heart problems. The most common heart problem, angina, is chest pains or tightness in the chest, feeling of indigestion, sometimes pain in the jaw, teeth or ear lobe, and numbness or tingling in any or all parts of the arm. Angina starts when the work of the heart is increased by exercise, stress, eating a big meal, or could happen even when someone is resting. It indicates that the blood flow to the heart has been temporary reduced, and actually is the heart muscle's call for help for more oxygen. It is for relief of this pain that many bypass operations are undertaken.

ARGUMENTS FOR AND AGAINST BYPASS SURGERY

FOR	AGAINST
Relieves the angina pains in 60 to 70% of patients not aided by drugs.	In one to four cases surgery is fatal.
Prolongs life if extensive obstruction exists in the left main artery.	In 5% the surgery precipitates a heart attack.
May improve life expectancy for angina patients with obstructions in three arteries who also have good function of the heart's main pumping chamber. Slow progressive build-up usually effects all areas rather evenly.	In patients with mild or no angina and one to three diseased arteries, there is no evidence that operation prevents heart attack or prolongs life.
	Within one year 20% of grafted arteries become closed and 7% of patients have reoccurence of angina.

In many leading medical centers there is a long waiting list, and patients must be prepared (except in emergency) to stand by for months for their place on the operating table. How would you like a business like that . . . a waiting list for a $20,000 service fee for about a half a day's work? Is it any wonder the medical profession cherishes this method of cure (?), and continues to sell patients on the possible temporary act of expectation and cure as the only method with no alternatives?

In the last few years there have been rumblings of discontent within medical circles.

With such a high volume of operations there are grafts that do not remain open and need a second or even a third operation. They grumble among themselves about the widespread use of an operation before risks and benefits are clearly explored. As a result of all this publicity, people are asking more questions.

Many patients, believe it or not, do not even consult their family doctor. The publicity is so great they make their own diagnosis and start looking for a cardiac surgeon. And now as interest and publicity grows, complaints mount, some hospitals and physicians are involved in a protective approach to this search for a broad range of candidates including those in the early stages of the disease who are "advised" to undergo the surgery "prophylatically". Many doctors with this approach even advocate doing diagnostic tests on patients who show no signs of pain but who have shown irregularities on cardiogram readings. If x-rays reveal any narrowing clues in the coronary area of these asymptomatic patients, they can recommend bypass surgery.

I can still see Jimmy Durante saying, "everybody is tryin to get into the act."

Patients who are relieved of chest pains may think that they have been miraculously cured of their heart disease. But they are wrong. In fact, the operation is merely a temporary pallative measure that treats symptoms for a limited time. The surgery **cannot cure artheriosclerosis**, which is a chronic progressive disease. Although some enthusiastic surgeons claim that it prolongs life and prevents heart attacks, this is yet to be demonstrated and there is evidence that the operation itself can cause significant damage to the heart. It involves long-term risk and actually accelerates the progression of artery disease. In some cases, the relief of symptoms is actually caused by a worsening of physical status . . . the surgery-induced death of the heart muscle, no longer in pain from inadequate oxygen supply.

As usual, all surgical results are suspect and biased, showing better survival rates. They are misleading because they use old data on medical treatments that are now considered improved since the use of drugs like Inderal, a vasodialator.

In fact, claims that the operation prolongs life have not been confirmed by the controlled studies, the AMA and FDA

BEFORE AND AFTER THE BYPASS

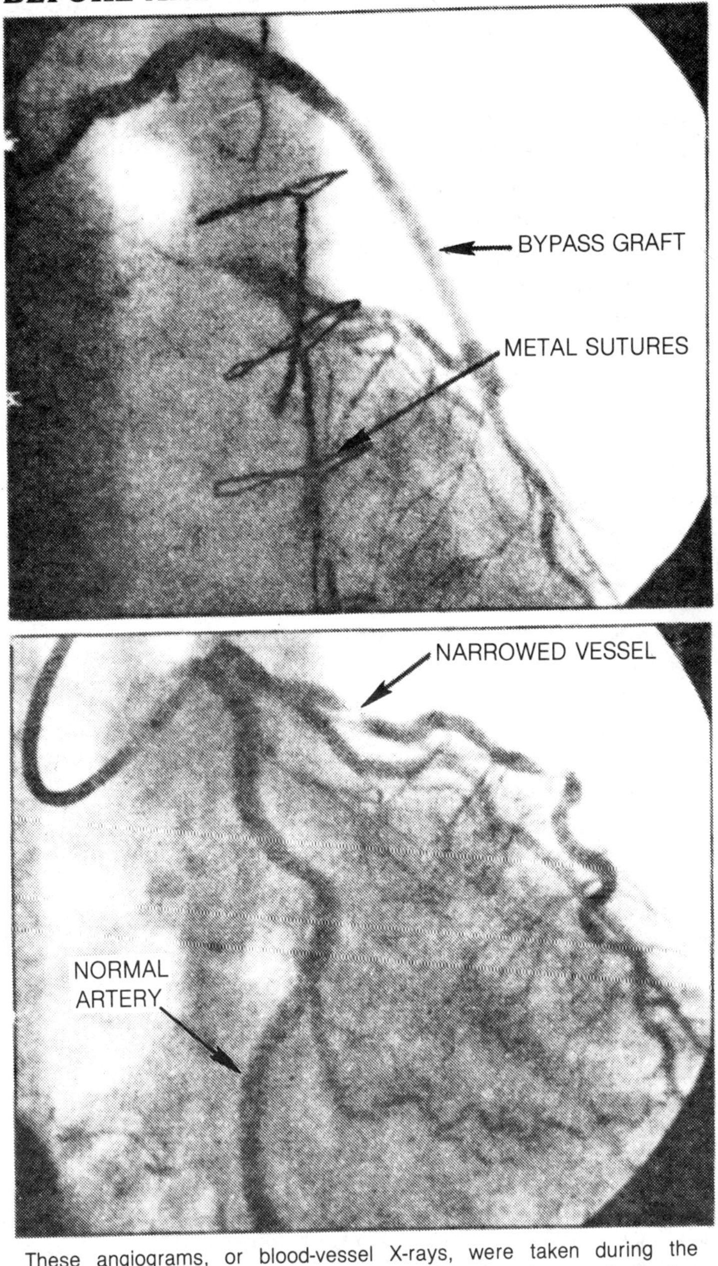

These angiograms, or blood-vessel X-rays, were taken during the catharization procedure. In the above photo is the same patient after bypass surgery with the sutures still showing; the new graft has bypasses the blocked area.

so often defensively refer. If your doctor brings up this point, ask to see the **"controlled studies"**.

A study by Dr. Wilbert Aranow of the University of California at Irvine that compared patients treated surgically to those treated with drugs showed no evidence of increased survival or lowered risk of heart attack as a result of surgery. Only one sub-group of very high-risk patients with chest pain has been shown to benefit from the surgery in terms of **survival** two years or more after the operation.

The operation involves some serious hazards. Stress, worry and fear cause some patients to die or have another heart attack right before or during surgery. Others have increased deterioration of the arteries that have been bypassed, a high rate of graft occlusions (which lead to a heart attack), or as reported, reappearance sometime later of severe chest pains because of the progressive nature of artery disease, possibly quickened by the surgery.

One of the risks is a surgically-induced heart attack. Many reports suggest that 5 to 40 percent of the patients experience a heart attack during or soon after the surgery. Many reports suggest that an average rate is about 15 to 25 percent.

If the patient comes through the operation safely there is no assurance that the grafts will remain open. There is documentation that the attachment of vein grafts causes significant increasing of disease in the vessels that receive the grafts. Then there is the possibility of grafts increasing the likelihood that new total occlusions will build up on either side of the graft.

As long as the grafts are patent, the closure of the arteries is no problem, but when the grafts themselves become occuluded later on, the patient is in a worse predictiment than before this surgery because he has now lost whatever arterial opening he previously had and faces the possibility of a greater risk of a coronary.

We have read the earlier hopes that bypass surgery would improve the function of the heart muscle; This is not so, nor has it been substantiated. Research reported by F.C. Spencer of New York University Medical Center showed that bypass grafting has little or no increased benefit on the function of the heart, particularly in patients who have already had a heart attack.

Of course, patients may get relief from pain and better tolerance for exercise even though there is no improvement in the heart. But even the one proven benefit of the relief of pain is only temporary. Even though artery disease is progressive, there is a possibility that surgery accelerates the problem and chest pains eventually reappear as you have already read. Dr. Paul Ticklenberg and his associates at Stanford Medical School reported that 40 percent of patients experienced chest pains 30 months after surgery than at nine months after surgery. (Forty-seven percent were unchanged and 13 percent felt better) We cannot lose sight of the progressive nature of the disease.

Patients and the general public are generally misled and their hopes held high by a more optimistic view they hear about on the surgery, more than support the facts. Patients are frequently told, for example, that the "mortality rates for this operation have been brought below two percent," even though their actual chances of dying in surgery may be higher, depending upon their own particular condition and where or who is doing the surgery. Many ethical surgeons resent some of the hospitals that boast the lowest mortality rate; some suspect that these hospitals use lower indications from surgery and operate on relatively healthy patients. The facts are sometimes twisted to suit the case.

MY PET COMPLAINT

There have never been any guidelines, laws, rules or requirements for reporting experiences with this surgery. It has never been restricted to research centers, even though its risks and benefits are still not fully shown. Rather it was quickly adopted for wide clinical use even before surgeons fully understood it. (What did Jimmie Durante say?) There is still no way of knowing who is doing it, for what reasons, and with what results. Dr. George E. Burch of Tulane University School of Medicine put it this way: "Imagine any capable cardiologist prescribing a pill that had never been subjected to double-blind studies, that might kill one out of ten patients, hurt 25 percent, produce pain and suffering in 100 percent, cost six thousand dollars to the patient, and never cure him! Not only would the cardiologist not prescribe the pill, but also the FDA would not allow the pill to reach the market and the public."

Yet the prestigeous AMA can abide by their own consciences without answering to anyone, in their own devious way. The FDA can approve or disprove any drug, but they hold little juristication over the AMA. Here again is why medical costs and health problems are out of hand.

You may ask why any of this controversy even among doctors has not reached the public. You are reading about many problems now. But if you know the inter-workings of doctors, their political effect, and their *"alleged code of ethics"* you would see that any strong statement against the

---

NEW STUDY SHOWS BYPASS HEART SURGERY IS OFTEN UNNECESSARY

A federally-sponsered study by the National Heart, Lung and Blood Institute says controversial coronary bypass surgery is not necessary in many cases in which it is now used.

Released last March at a meeting of the American College of Cardiology, the report said investigators found that mortality is low, and equal, for each type of treatment; that heart attacks occur more often after surgery, and that angina pain persists more after drug treatment than surgery.

In the four-year study, doctors at eight medical centers tested 288 patients of whom 147 received intensive drug therapy, and 141 submitted to bypass surgery.

In the medically-treated group, the death rate in the hospital was 4.1%, and for the surgical patients it was 5.2%. During hospitalization, 18% of the bypass patients suffered heart attacks as compared with 10% in the medically-treated group.

Fifteen percent of the surgery patients reported at least one incident of posthospital angina chest pain, as compared with 45% of the medical group. (Angina is chest pain caused when the heart muscle fails to get enough oxygen, usually because one or more of major blood vessel is constricted or blocked by fatty deposits).

Dr. Michael B. Mock, the Institute's project officer, told Associated Press it is estimated that as many as 70,000 bypass operations are performed each year in this country. At the cost of $10,000 to $15,000, critics say surgery is overused because it is profitable.

Dr. Mock said the data showed that delaying surgical treatment had "no effect on morality, and this means that two-thirds of the medical group was spared surgery."

A "small percentage" of unstable angina patients require immediate surgery, he said the study showed, but "many others could wait." (Angina is called unstable when first noticed, or if there is a changing pattern of pain in an existing condition).

NATIONAL HEALTH FEDERATION BULLETIN — FEBRUARY 1980

Medicare Pays for Expensive Heart Transplants, But Not Chelation

Medical "experts" in the U.S. Public Health Service, agreeing with Stanford Medical Center that heart transplants no longer are "experimental," consented in November to pay for the transplants —but only those performed at Stanford because it has acheived "a high rate of success by carefully selecting patients and vigorously treating the transplant patient for rejection of the donor heart."

Oakland Blue Cross, which handles Medicare claims in northern California, had been paying for the transplants by error. Payments were cut off in May, after which Stanford Medical Center officials presented evidence persuading the government that the procedure is "not experimental."

Average cost of a transplant is $130,000. Stanford has been doing about 24 a year. The survival record: 70% of those receiving a new heart live "at least one year, 50% at least five years."

Stanford's transplant team estimates that 75,000 Americans a year could benifit from the surgery, which at present costs would be about $10 billion annually.

Medicare payments are made only for surgery or treatment "considered standard medical practice."

Because of that criterion, such treatment as chelation is not covered.

(If a $130,000 heart transplant is covered by Medicare, why not chelation therapy, which costs only a fraction of that amount, and survival factor is at least as good, probably considerably higher? It is valuable as a preventive measure against heart seizure and stroke. Ed.)

NATIONAL HEALTH FEDERATION BULLETIN — FEBRUARY 1980

---

operation would likely lead to angry words from many of their own colleagues. One research cardiologist privately expressed his opinion that 80 percent of bypass operations are "worthless" apart from the temporary relief of symptoms (angina) and said this was a very sensitive area in medicine.

It wasn't many years ago, before bypass surgery gained popularity, the yearly AMA presidential address to organizations of thoracic surgeons asked the group to restrict its production of new members. There were too many surgeons coming out of training and not enough business for them. Much of their business was disappearing because of advances in the various heart disease categories. But the explosion of artery surgery had these same surgeons find a new and unlimited source of patients, a new *"windfall"* better than before.

A busy cardiac surgeon can easily earn over a half million dollars a year doing this surgery. There is a financial incentive for cardiologists to recommend bypass surgery. They are paid much more money to perform post-operative and pre-operative procedures than to manage patients with non-surgical therapies. So my cardiologist or yours can recommend surgery in order to keep his own practice busy.

Cardiologists have a personal and financial interest in referring patients to surgeons working in their own hospitals however they might evaluate the surgeon's skills. Hospitals and physicians' colleagues systematically overlook medical errors and discrepancies and because there are no structures for monitoring incompetence; the only time incompetence gets widely exposed is when there is public scandal. In the case of some surgery the evidence is buried with the patient.

In 1969, the Intersociety Commission for Heart Disease Resources was convened by various medical and surgical associations in a very noble effort to issue guidelines about what resources such as personnel and equipment a hospital should have in order for that facility to properly undertake heart surgery. The same problems arise today as "bypass qualification" is questioned. When asked, by interviewer, Marcia Millman, one cardiac surgeon who served on the committee, why there were no controlled studies of bypass surgery before it was widely used, and why all hospitals were allowed to perform it even though they fall short of the ICHD guidelines, he said, "Well, you could say that we sacrifice people, and some people die; but people are dying off like flies anyway. They are dying of heart attacks by the millions. And you could say there are too many people anyway."

There is talk among some physicians for an equivalent of the FDA for surgery. I believe the same powerful force that dominates surgery practice is also likely to dominate any committee set up to regulate it.

(Reprinted in part from 9/13/76 NEW WEST as adapted before publication of the forthcoming book THE UNKINDEST CUT by Marcia Millman, Assistant Professor of Sociology, University of California, Santa Cruz. Published by William Morrow Company N.Y. 1977.)

ADDENDUM

In medicine FOR LAYMAN on the subject of HEART ATTACKS reprinted 5/80 by U.S.H.E.W. by the Public Health Service and National Institute of Health on page 16 & 17, there appears this comment. "However, there is no evidence yet that coronary bypass surgery improves the function of the left ventricule or that it makes the heart pump better. In fact, there is some evidence that the bypass surgery may actually decrease efficiency. Clinical investigations are now trying to determine whether bypass surgery improves or impairs heart function and whether it increases a patients life expectancy." Later it goes on to say this makes it important to us to find out whether we are improving the patients outlook and prognosis as well as relieving pain." Here is proof published by our own government and authored by Dr. Robert I. Levy, Director, National Heart, Lung and Blood Institute.

Here is an admission of doubt of importance to patients from the very highest of places. The one billion cost is now two billion apparently, the insurance industry supports medicare and subsidizes the surgery. And it seems that the government and science should determine once and for all the beneficial status of bypass surgery and chelation therapy. There is a double standard involved here. The AMA and conventional medicine influences government without testing the procedure, to the tune of two billion dollars a year in payments for an admittedly questionable surgical procedure. While the same political influence prevents the administration and payment, for chelation therapy that is much safer, more thorough and less costly. And thus dear reader do we again see the power that conventional medicine holds over the government and the lives of all people.

SUMMARY THOUGHT!

Seeing and believing has changed into a doubtful state of the mind because of the power of the printed word and television. When feelings and emotions, or a human life are involved . . . buyer beware.

Chapter Thirteen
DOCTORS OF DECEIT

"All our knowledge merely helps us die a more painful death than animals who know nothing."

. . . Maurice Maeterlinck

The American Medical Association (AMA) is motivated by ignorance, greed and arrogance in their quest to stifle chelation therapy.

Here's what some heart patients are told by various physicians:

- "No matter what we do, the situation is dismal."
- "Go home, make your will; put your house in order."
- There are no alternatives; we have done all that we can." (referring to bypass surgery)
- "There is no hope of success; there is no guarantee, and no alterantive."
- "I wouldn't make any long-term investments. You're sitting on a powder key. You could go at any moment."
- "Make her comfortable and she will slowly slip away."

These physicians, regardless of their personal opinions, education, beliefs or motivations, are breaking their Hypocratic Oath they took upon receiving their medical degree. These despairing statements should hardly be needed if the physician would condescend to administer chelation therapy, and modify their selfish motives.

The AMA whose membership has dwindled to representing only 38 percent of organized physicians are put under fire here as the most powerful organized group in the Country. In as much as 38 percent is not representative of all licensed physicians, this writer believes the 38 percent has indicated to be powerful enought to represent a much larger

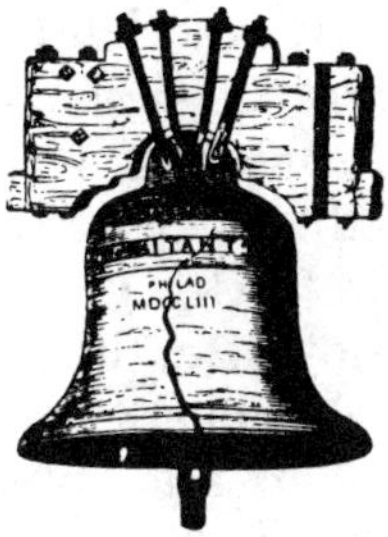

The Constitution of this Republic
should make special provision
for MEDICAL SCIENCE.
To restrict the art of healing
to one class
will constitute
the bastile of Medical Science.
All such laws
are un-American
and despotic.

Benjamin Rush, Physician
Signer of the
Declaration of Independence

segment of the profession who do hold and practice similar beliefs and have been educated to practice in a similiar way as the AMA membership. Accordingly this is not an indictment of all practical physicians.

It appears that the AMA has set itself up as a despot that would attempt to dictate to you what is best from a health standpoint for your body. They attempt to legislate almost every competative idea out of existance. For instance chiropractors are the top of their "HIT" list. Then there is the vurnable members of AAMP's exposed to publicity from their exciting treatments, are harassed in devious legal ways. Such legal defense for this legal harassment always ends up in appeals, making such defense expensive. The devious part is that it is hoped the harassed physician's morale, fortitude and financial means will be broken down in eventual surrender.

The AMA effort to attempt to destroy chiropractic and chelation therapy is a threat to our rights of freedom to choose our own health therapy. As consumers, we must not be limited to those health practicioners and treatments approved by the AMA. History reveals they have put their own self-interest before their patients welfare.

Robert Berko, editor of Caveat Emptor Bulletin, declared in an editorial title, "Can We Afford The AMA Monopoly?" states: "Study after study will show that 30 percent or more of surgical procedures are unnecessary. This has cost us billions of dollars and at least 16,000 deaths each year. The medical profession is so contaminated by these surgical butchers that unions and insurance companies now are willing to pay for "second opinions" to stop this carnage and murder. And yet, the medical establishment does very little to cleanse itself; in fact, it defends its butchers."

A surgeon once said that surgeons themselves joke that if any of their breed were asked to name the three greatest surgeons in the world, he would be hard-pressed to name the other two.

Each year hundreds of qualified applicants are turned away from the doors of our medical schools. How this happends is not an accident. This is a "control" situation by the AMA policy boards. According to a report released earlier in 1980 by President Carter's Council on Wage and Price Stability, "There is considerable evidence that for much of this century, organized medicine has successfully restricted entry into the medical profession, primarily through its control of state licensing processes and the system of medical education."

Even their own doctors comment that they place more emphasis on treating the symptoms than preventing or curing the disease.

Senator Edward Kennedy said July 1970, "The organization of health services is still in shambles. Why? Because the AMA and its friends in the health insurance industry have stood in the way of every major step toward an efficient, effective, affordable health care system for the American people.

"Instead of the scientific and public professional organization it was founded as, the AMA has turned into a propaganda organ purveying 'medical politics' for deceiving the Congress, the people, and the doctors of America themselves."

National Health Expenditures:
1960 to 1978

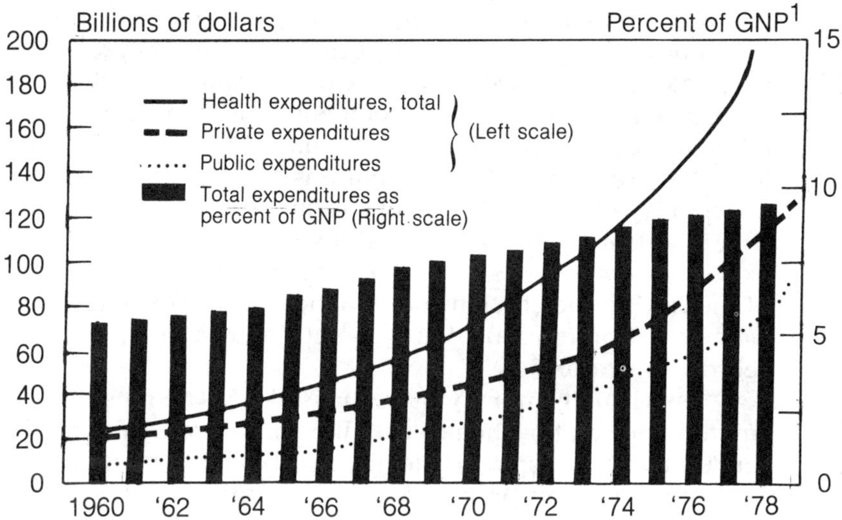

[1]Gross national product.
Source: Chart prepared by U.S. Bureau of Census.
Data from U.S. Health Care Financing Administration.

The largest and richest lobby in Washington is maintained by the AMA. Figures available for 1965 show, according to **Health Rights News** of August 1969, in that year alone the AMA lobby spent $1.1 million . . . ten times more than was spent by the second largest, that of the AFL-CIO. It is noteworthy that at that time, the total AMA budget was over twenty million dollars, 45 percent of this sum derived from advertising in the AMA publications by drug companies and medical suppliers.

Heres an example of the AMA biting the government hand that feed it. The AMA has lobbied and brought the level of **government financed** revenues of medical schools to almost 50 percent. There is a long list of proposals that at one time or another were vigorously, but as it turned out, vainly opposed by the AMA. A listing of the important legislation that the AMA unsuccessfully tried to kill includes: child labor laws; minimum wage laws; the 40-hour week; Medicare; Medicaid; mass X-ray screening for chest diseases like TB and lung cancer; government-sponsored VD clinics; compulsory reporting of cummunicable diseases; and many more.

U.S. expenditures for health needs are greater than in any other nation (140 billion dollars in 1976), and readers might be entitled to think that at this high cost they get both the most and the best medical care possible. If delivery of medical care were what management consultants call "cost efficient" we would be first among nations.

But we are not. Thirteen nations rank ahead of us in life expectancy of males; 18 nations rank ahead of us in preventing infant mortality; and 7 nations rank ahead of us in life expectancy of females. Thus, if life itself is used as a standard of measuring the efficiency of U.S. health care expenditures, we as a nation must be doing something wrong, and should reorder our priorities.

As virtually monopolists, the AMA has **the** most powerful influence on how health care innovations are undertaken and treated . . . in spite of the huge portion of our national income that is spent on health care, the United States has an unfortunate standing in heart disease epidemic in the early 1970s.

1971 CORONARY THROMBOSIS DEATH RATE BY COUNTRY
(per 100,000 population)

Country	**Rate**
Finland	224.7
U.S.A.	211.8
Australia	204.6
Canada	187.4
United Kingdom	140.9
Netherlands	106.9
West Germany	102.3
Austria	88.6
Italy	78.9
Switzerland	75.9
Sweden	74.7
France	41.7
Japan	39.1

The average family is spending 13 percent of its income on health care. And, this cost is rising faster than the inflation rate and will soon overcome us, unless something is done.

This sector of our economy seems to be running out of control and no one seems to know how to stop it. Economists and government officials are worried about the situation, so much so that insurance companies are now endorsing second opinions before surgery.

In fact, at a recent conference, HEW Secretary Joseph Califano and Senator Edward Kennedy both expressed concern that unless we can keep the present health delivery establishment from continuing this escalation of costs, it will undermine our whole financial structure. It is happening . . . now.

Why is this? It is in a great measure because our medical-oriented system is a monopoly, controlled and manipulated by the AMA.

The AMA has long been known as one of the most conservative bodies in the country. It is a prestigious organization staffed by brilliant people who are able to influence a great majority of people in any cause they are involved in.

Through a long-term calculated program of propaganda and judicious use of political contributors, the AMA has **gained control** of colleges, government agencies, state medical boards, hospitals, health insurers, and other health professionals.

Conditions have now reached a point where all these factors have been put together to produce well above average income for medical doctors. They can charge (and get) almost any fee. It is believed the aim of the AMA is not to provide better health care but to gain better income for doctors. Medical doctors earn much more than others with the same years of education. M.D.s earning $500,000. a year are not unusual.

The supply of competitors within the medical profession is controlled **by limiting** the number of medical school graduates and **by limiting** the services that can be performed by nurses, technicians, and other medical personnel.

The competition from practitioners of other health disciplines is kept under control by villification and manipulation of legislators, medical boards, and insurance carriers.

The doctor supply increased somewhat during the

1960s due more to immigration of foreign doctors into the United States than to any reversal in the policies of the AMA.

In the area of medical diagnosis the picture is gloomy. A 1967 paper by the U.S. Public Health Service and consultant, Barkey S. Sanders, Ph.D., which examined the results of many other studies, showed that a patient electing to go to a doctor with some unknown ailment has only a one to five chance of receiving a proper diagnosis of his illness. The studies cited by Sanders revealed, too, that unknown disease is many times manifested, despite the fact that people make five visits on average to a doctor each year. And within a then recent two-year period, only 19 percent of the people failed to see a doctor. Dr. Sanders found that "only 40 percent of all human ailments are found and labeled by doctors, and 60 percent are missed. Of those diseases that are presumed to be found, one-half are diagnosed in error."

The National Federation of State Medical Boards estimated in 1976 that doctors making up five percent of the nation's total (16,000 doctors) are literally unfit to practice medicine, even though such numbers treat an estimated 7.5 million patients a year and may account for many thousands of needless deaths and injuries.

"In 1976, the House Oversight and Investigations Subcommittee released a report saying approximately 2.4 million unnecessary surgeries were performed in the United States in 1974 alone. The subcommittee estimated that this cost 11,900 deaths a year. Later, new investigations by the subcommittee found the deplorable situation virtually unchanged."

"This knife-happy approach of medicine, razor sharp to the needs of these doctors and awfully dull in dealing with the problem of patients, seems unaffected by publicity and is very set in its ways. Consequently, without an uproar of scandalous headlines, business will go on "as usual".

There are few who would disagree that our health care industry is one of the most costly in the western world. Also that there is need for change.

Every year about 30,000 Americans receive drugs their doctors prescribe, and die as a result. At least ten times as many of these patients are subjected to life-threatening and oft-times permanent side-effects." So ends Berkos editorial comment.

"That a problem of preventable adverse drug reaction exists cannot be denied," said Dr. John C. Ballin, Director of the AMA's Department of Drugs. He said the literature is loaded with references to the prescribing of the inaccurate or wrong drugs, or wrong dose, to unlikely drug reactions, or just to the prescribing of a drug when none was actually needed.

Dr. Sidney Wolfe of the Health Research Group, a consumer advocacy organization affiliated with Ralph Nader, estimates, on the basis of published data, that in 22 percent of the cases, antibiotic treatments in hospitals are unnecessary. With the fatal reactions that occur with these drugs, Dr. Wolfe figured with the annual rate of fatal reactions that more than 10,000 patients could have been spared an ordeal if the drugs were omitted from treatment.

Dr. William R. McCabe, an infectious disease expert at Boston University Medical School, reported in the **New England Journal of Medicine** that the incidence of infections may now be as high as one percent of all patients admitted to hospitals. Such superinfection can occur when patients are given broad spectrum antibiotics that kill a wide range of organisms. Dr. McCabe estimates there are 100,000 deaths a year from superinfection.

Various other medical experts have estimated that up to one-half of the antibiotics administered in hospitals are not really necessary, and that about the same percentage of deaths due to gram-negative superinfection could be prevented by more intelligent use of antibiotics.

We hear about "adverse reactions" that we thought not too long ago were too rare to be mentioned. Today we read they occur by the tens of thousands each day. They actually kill more victims than some types of cancer, and they are listed in the top ten causes of hospitalization. But as is usually the case, the medical associations just deny that there is misuse, over-prescribing or any problem at all.

We see adverse drug problems in the news. The obvious problem of drug reaction is a health menace, so alarming the news has brought investigations, or inquiries are planned.

And what can we say about drug prices? How high is too high? . . . V.D. Mattia, M.D., President of Hoffman La Roache, in 1969 said, "I can't honestly say that drug prices are cheap. I think they are reasonable only for those who can afford to pay the price."

"It is significant to note," George Squibb once testified, "that the industries' pricing policies and practices have not only brought sharp criticism from those in the academic, press, and legislature circles outside the pharmacy and medical professions, but also from those within those professions." Squibb came down hard on the industry when he declared that friendly and opponents alike point with alarm, shame, disgust, distrust and perplexity, and what is certain a situation hard to justify, chaotic, shortsighted and stupid.

In all due respect to an industry that has researched and brought thousands of new drugs to the market, and saved and prolonged many thousands of lives, it now suffers from gross overexposure of its products through its doctor dispensers. While it does not seem so, the drug industry basically has but one customer who prescribes the drugs . . . the physician. While you cannot blame them for supporting their one customer, their methods, motives and high prices seem to be a result of these physician motives they foster. Doing business with an unregulated monopoly such as the AMA, could be the root of the overall problem with the drug industry.

The AMA, the FDA, and the drug industry are a solid triangle of strength . . . the center of the triangle is filled with solid gold dollars to keep it strong, (product advertising in the *AMA Journal*) spawned by the drug industry, spilled over into the AMA coffers, and to the bureaucracy support of the FDA.

The drug industry practically supports the **AMA Journal** 100 percent with its advertising for drugs. If no advertising appeared on a non-profitable drug, a doctor would possibly not want to prescribe the drug, thinking it is not recommended anymore, as it is not advertised in the **Journal.** He is more likely to read the drug advertising sales message in the **Journal** than he is the warning of contra-indications on the small paper insertion packed with the drug.

In 1968 the HEW task force devised this definition of rational prescribing: "The right drug for the right patient, at the right time, in the right amounts, and with due consideration of relative costs." It seems that definitions are one thing, but the AMA knows they control the entire situation.

At the time, leading clinicians and medical educators were expressing their grave concern for the then serious problem of prescribing drugs. "It is my belief," said Dr. Jan Koch-Weser of Harvard, "that lack of knowledge in the proper therapeutic use of drugs is perhaps the greatest deficiency of the average American physician today."

Naturally, from such comments we expect excuses, counter claims and pushing the blame on the pharmacologists, who have criticized their counterparts.

I wonder how long the AMA can defend its long-cherished independence and especially the physician's individual freedom to prescribe drugs as he alone sees fit? There is no law, license or decree for doctors to follow. He can choose and use any drug in any way he cares to, no matter how careless or knowledgable he may or may not be on drugs, or how he keeps up-to-date on drug education.

This seems to be the area where basic blame can be placed. The organized medical profession's system or theory in treating symptoms rather than relying on finding a cure actually places the burden on the physician to prescribe to his individual ability and discretion.

Dr. Arnold Relman, one of the medical worlds most respected figures and editor of the Nation's most respected medical publication, the New England Journal of Medicine, in the December 22, 1980 issue made a plea to physicians to divest themselves of profit-making medical businesses earning billions of dollars.

Dr. Relman remarked that the AMA should declare it unethical for a doctor to derive any income from health care except his own services. He pointed out they have become a part of *'ownership of for-profit hospitals'*, nursing homes, kidney dialysis businesses, laboratories, pain clinics and many other health support firms. It was estimated that perhaps a third of the 240 billion dollar a year health care industry is in private hands.

Dr. Relman remarked that this money-making industrial complex and doctors financial interest in it are growing, and unless doctors give it up, the public will lose confidence in them as honest disinterested representatives of their patients best interests.

Moreover, Relman said, doctors will be lending themselves to a new *vested interest* lobby affecting the nation's laws. Already the doctor-controlled kidney dialysis industry 'blunted the force' of the new law that could have moved thousands of patients from private clinics to cheaper home dialysis.

As another example of potential conflict between a doctor's financial interest and his patient's welfare, Relman quoted from a brochure published by Brookwood Health Services of Birmingham, Alabama, one of the many corporations that operate investor-owned hospitals. The firm said the brochure *views each physician as a business partner,* and because to this he said, it recruits young physicians and subsidizes their start.

Of course there was rebuttal such as AMA officials who admitted that this should not happen and remarked that doctors should not be on "both sides of the fence". (End of defense)

Along the same lines I read in the St. Petersburg times the other day that complaints are surfacing on the high charges that doctors are marking-up laboratory fees. These tests are usually farmed out to private specialty labs. (many owned by the doctors) The large number of complaints averaged a 101 percent mark-up on the doctors' costs. This is according to an unpublished report by the General Accounting Office and written in the Times.

In the fast-growing sun belt areas, the happy hunting grounds for doctors, advertising is appearing keyed to price and accessability of doctors. Privately operated medical clinics are starting to appear in large shopping centers where minor emergencies and medical services can be performed. The long hours and staffing are designed to catch the masses.

I would not be surprised to see Sears and Wards get into the act also. They have opened eye examinations by financing complete examination rooms for optometrists, to compliment their optical business. They already have complete dental clinics operating in some locations. All this to take advantage of the convenience of the monthly charge-all credit card and insure the store of a better return on its reputation.

But none of these innovations worry me as much as the AMA effort to lobby against their own sins and shortcomings.

They have the power and the money to buy their way out of most any trouble they may encounter.

In 1970, both claims and malpractice rates shot sky high. Many insurance companies quit the business, forcing doctors and hospital groups in some areas to organize their own malpractice insurance companies.

Today, 10 years later we have a new surge of malpractice suits amounting to 10 billion dollars yearly. Hospitals operate as businesses for profit pay two-thirds of these insurance costs and 75 percent of lawsuits arising from treatments within such hospitals. Even the remaining 25 percent of doctor blamed costs is a significant factor.

PROSPECTIVE, the Blue Cross/Blue Shield magazine reports that big insurance companies who have been writing this business for years, suffered a loss of 150 million dollars in underwriting in 1979. 1980 figures are expected to surge even higher. There is now concern about the long term viability of the new doctor/hospital owned malpractice insurance carriers.

The Perspective article states that malpractice suits and the practice of "defensive medicine" probably are costing 10 billion dollars a year. Defensive medicine means ordering many expensive tests and other procedures designed more to protect the doctors and hospitals from technical charges of negligence, than because they are necessary in treating the patient.

A book by Thomas R. Mulroy, HOSPITAL LIABILITY REVISITED, Inquiry Books, Chicago, seems to have frightened the health-care industry considerably because it called attention to a hitherto largely ignored 1975 New Jersey court decision. Known as the Colerto Decision, it rules that the administration and trustees of hospitals and all the doctors on its professional staff could be held liable along with the hospital in a case of malpractice. The court in effect, accepted the plaintiff's argument that the entire administration and staff of a hospital had to be aware of the facts if a surgeon was allowed to perform an operation for which he was not competent and, therefore, must share in the liability. Author Mulroy predicts that this doctrine will take root and warns doctors and hospital administrators that the only defense against legal doctrine is better standards of patient care.

And one last thought. When you skinned your knee as a child you never wondered whether it would get better or not. You just knew the bleeding would stop all by itself, a scab would form, and within a few days your knee would be like new again. As you grew older you were soon taught that to get better when you are sick or hurt, you have to see a doctor and get some "medicine". So once again the "medical arts" is passed on to another generation without realizing it. You somehow lost that youthful "blind faith" in the body's healing system.

From the moment we were conceived, we were blessed with the most perfect and intricate systems a living organism has ever known. All living organisms are self-constructing, self defending, self-maintaining and self-repairing. There is no other organism to depend on for these functions. It does not need to be prodded or coaxed into action by artificial or outside means, normally. The system is automatically activated in the event of illness or injury.

We should all take the time for our own assumption of responsibility and well being so we can change our habits and lifestyles to allow this self-renewal to happen to all of us.

"I firmly believe that if the whole materia medica, as now used, could be sunk to the bottom of the sea, it would be better for mankind and all the worse for the fishes." So said Dr. Oliver Wendall Holmes at an address before the Massachusetts Medical Society in 1860.

SUMMARY THOUGHT!

Blessed are the pure in thoughts, for they shall pay their doctor homage. Blessed are the ill advised for they shall pay their doctor's high fees. Blessed are the believers as they shall reach the hospital. Blessed are the poor in spirit as they shall be rewarded with despair and suffering. Blessed are the faithful for they shall be disillusioned.

Chapter Fourteen
"STAYING SLIM AND THE NO-NO FAT"

"Most people eat as though they were fattening themselves for the market."

. . . Edgar W. Howe

NOTE: This is a report on fat two ways; as added weight in body tissue and as food consumed in our diets. This and the next chapter show alternatives to weight control that seem to rate meritorious mention. This is not expert medical opinion, even though such weight loss methods are already popular and proven methods for losing weight. Any popular weight loss program will tell you to seek preliminary medical help. I say, seek experienced professionals in nutrition and preventive medicine.

This fat subject matter is the most important cause of heart disease. Fat affects my health in a major way. Anyone concerned with overweight as I am, should take this subject very seriously.

Fat is one nutrient that has the deck stacked against it. Overweight, obesity, diet related fat are blamed on almost every problem of health. On symptoms of heart disease there is a direct relationship with too much fat or overweight. Heart attack and death statistics are overwhelming on overweight people.

AMERICANS HAVE A LOVE AFFAIR WITH FAT! . . . TO THEIR EVENTUAL SORROW.

Doctors at the prestigious Cleveland Clinic are calling it JUNK FOOD DISEASE. A study authored by Dr. Derrick Lonsdale, head of the Biochemical Genetics Section at the Clinic, was published recently in the *American Journal of Clinical Nutrition.*

The study was aimed at American youngsters and teenagers, among whom the problem is becoming a serious health hazard. Here's the danger that is caused by the so called Junk Food Disease:

✓ There's a serious deficiency of vitamin B-1 that causes youngsters to become aggressive, irritable, with personality changes, loss of sleep or frightening dreams.

✓ Candy, french fries, potato chips and soda pop head the list of dangerous common diets.

✓ The study found a pattern of symptoms likened to old fashioned Beriberi, common in Southeast Asia years ago and caused by a deficiency in thiamine or vitamin B-1.

✓ The patients in the study had diets consisting of what Dr. Lonsdale called "naked calories" or lacking in vitmains and minerals.

The study concluded that the responsibility rests with the parents to provide a proper diet by substituting fresh fruits for snacks, fresh fruit juice for soda pop and by eating a one-a-day vitamin to the diet. Then change the youngsters' eating habits. I remind you that it is at this age and under these eating habits that the seed is planed for future occlusive artery disease. The insidious buildup starts.

The fat in the long-time obese person may become dilated, flabby and weak as it becomes infiltrated with fat deposits that continues to reduce its efficiency. Many times enlargement occurs while thickening of its muscular wall takes place as a compensatory effect for the excess load carried. Rarely can this *"fat type" of heart be operated on at all.*

Coronary thrombosis, or occlusion, is more likely to occur in obese persons. Once the coronary occurs, the life expectancy and ability to carry normal activity is greatly reduced. So isn't it better to keep thin, and be more ensured.

It is common information that the pulse is faster in obese people. This is due to the heart's effort to compensate for the strain of a continuously present excess load. High blood pressure tends to develop more often in obese people, and it is noted that the blood pressure drop backward toward normal on reduction of excess weight.

Intake of fats from our diets is a much discussed subject and of concern to everyone today because there exists a relationship between abnormal blood liquid levels (fat) and heart and vascular disease.

FAT AND THE HEART

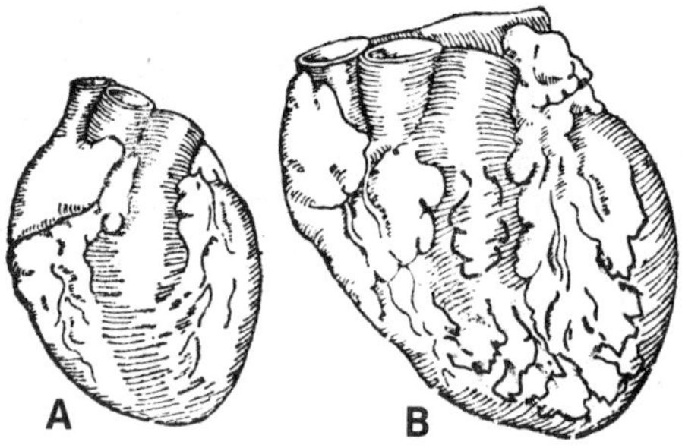

A = Normal Heart. *B* = Enlarged Heart (with flabby deposits of fat surrounding the muscle tissue). Obesity causes the fat deposits between the ventricles.

While such a relationship exists, the role of dietary fat is not fully understood as yet. Accordingly, you will find differences of opinion as to amount and type of fat. Dietary cholesterol, high serum cholesterol and fatty acids are also misunderstood. Some relate to internal metabolism rather than from what we eat. Here is where medical experience in diet and nutrition is so important to everyone.

Many of the medical experts I have talked to on the subject of nutrition and diet feel that Dr. Robert Atkins is a very knowledgeable expert on such problems. His first book is a best seller, *Dr. Atkins Diet Revolution* (Bantam Books) and his latest scientific effort, *Dr. Atkins Nutritional Breakthrough*, are worth reading and the most practical, for those who earnestly wish to lose weight. Dr. Atkins states, "It isn't the number of calories, it is the kind of calories that count."

In this first book you will read that the AMA instigated charges against Dr. Atkins. There developed widespread discussion and controversy on criticism of his diet ideas. This occurred in 1973 and provoked a hearing of the U.S. Senate Select Committee on Nutrition and Human Needs. Some committee members were even swayed by the adverse publicity generated. The charges were that the diet may be adverse to the dieter's health.

While Dr. Atkins completely answered the charges before the committee, the actual testimony is contained in the back of his book. It is interesting and educational. While Dr. Atkins did not avoid the harrassment and ridicule, he gained in stature from his defense of his popular diet. It is believed that the new book, *Nutritional Breakthrough,* will eventually be used as reference in the control of our health care in the future.

Dr. Atkins, in short, suggests a no or low carbohydrate diet . . . eat all you wish but not carbohydrates. He says we are victims of carbohydrate poisoning which is similar to naked or empty calories. But who among us argue with a very successful best seller? Who could argue with: eat all you wish of most any food except carbohydrates? Who could argue with not eating sweets, starches or certain saturated fats and adding, if they bring about better health and a loss of weight?

Fat is calories in concentrated form, and while it is a nutrient, it is the most fatting nutrient we eat. For instance, one gram of fat gives us nine calories, and one gram of carbohydrates gives us only four calories. There is no doubt that you really have to cut down on fat consumption to keep thin or lose weight.

We should all know that polyunsaturated fats, the good fats, are beneficial fats in our diet for the life of the cell and are classified as "oils." While the saturated fats, the bad fats, are the problem fats and are classified as "solids". This identification is related to what fats do inside your body. But we only need one to two percent of polyunsaturated fats in our diet anyway, and none of the saturated fats . . . so we really don't need much fat at all. (Look down at your stomach and see.)

What we need to talk about is "animal fats" that are saturated fats. These are the real enemies. We are supposed to eat "cholesterol-lowing" polyunsaturated fats, but the *animal fats* are the fats we really *do not need.*

My dear wife, and I am sure many of you, are victims of our own (bad) habits. Who started that idea that you must eat meat almost every meal? I really have trouble breaking my wife of this habit . . . but inflation (has some good points) and the high cost of meat, helps her cut down somewhat. I have her trained to chicken, fish and meat in order of importance.

Ninety-eight percent of all the fats we eat are not needed, I am told, from a nutritional standpoint. Less than a tablespoon is needed daily and this is of course polyunsaturated fat. The average person eats eight times more fat than that and that is why there are fat unhealthy people. So I cut off the fat around the slice of ham, or trim the fat off a steak because I can see the fat. But I eat the rest of the meat where I cannot see the hidden fat between the grains, which is called marbling. Worse yet, the more marbling, the more tender the steak.

A synthetic fat is a laboratory concoction usually made from cheap vegetable oil (cottonseed or coconut oil) by a process called hydrogenation. It is the food processing industries' answer to profits. The vegetable oil is processed with a metal catalyst and hydrogen and the original oil is destroyed and a new component takes its place. Vitamins and minerals are lost in the process. The dark substance is bleached to an attractive white color. It ends up tasteless and foodless as a widely-used synthetic hydrogenated fat. The nutritional value is absolutely zero except for the added calories, called empty calories.

Synthetic fats and chemicals are taken into our bodies one way or another. These are very hard to get rid of. They steal the essential enzymes, vitamins, and minerals from other areas of metabolism in order to be metabolized out of the body. So, as a result, we find nutritional deficiencies suchas vitamins in the B-complex class and Vitamin E, enzymes, and minerals. So they all have to be replaced by more vitamins, minerals, and enzymes themselves. This is the problem of junk foods and processed foods.

So look out for partially or hydrogenated fats. This fancy word means trouble. Many brands of margarine, salad oils, mayonnaise, snack foods, and processed foods contain these substances. And, if you think sweets are just a source of sugar, you are mistaken. Milk chocolate, ice cream, baked goods, to mention some, have large amounts of these fats in them. Mass-produced peanut butter is high in hydrogenated or partly-hardened oils and fats. Natural peanut butter has no hydrogenated fats to add to your weight.

So the only thing to do is eat less fats, take the B-complex vitamins including Biotin, take Vitamin E, and remember the enzymes that play a part in digesting foods, including the fats.

Lecithin has been shown to lower the concentration of cholesterol and other fats in the blood that may lead to heart disease. The cholesterol levels in the blood of middle-aged men is a powerful pre-indication of which men will get heart disease and which men will die from it. Also, levels of triglycerides (other fats) are higher in people suffering from clogged arteries.

Soybean lecithin is a natural food product that is a lipid (fat) reducing agent. Lecithin also appears naturally in egg yolks and liver in large amounts.

Fats are also found in cheese, deep-fried foods, nuts, chocolate, creamed soups, and the higher the quality of ice cream the higher the butterfat content, as in most dairy products. Luncheon meats and bacon not only are high in fats but they have salts added in quantity to "cure" the food. Take coffee whiteners that substitute for coffee creams; look at the contents on the label. They may be worse fats than the butterfat in regular coffee cream.

Restaurant menus today many times come from not the restaurant itself but from a commercially-prepared or processed food kitchen, so as to broaden the menu. Microwave ovens go handily with processed foods and are a prerequisite in most restaurants and fast food chains. You can tell the menu is processed from the creamed names, the gravy names, the au gratin and the ala mode names. There are also marinated and casserole dishes processed. Doesn't it seem better to look for poached, pickled, garden fresh, in broth, in tomato sauce, or in its own juices as clues to better restaurant eating? And of course, always order food broiled or baked rather than deep fried or even pan fried.

I also have found out that to make matters worse in the fat war, fats that are heated to high temperatures (200 degrees F.) has a known effect on artheriosclerosis as tested on animals in the laboratory. Actually, some fats turn almost to solids when these oils separate from the heating developed in the cooking. And who wants that?

Measured facts reveal every pound of fat in our bodies contains almost five thousand feet of blood vessels. (Read that again.) If you have five pounds excess fat, your heart must push the blood through about 25 extra miles of blood vessels every half second. For any normal heart even, this places a needless strain that can be prevented by proper diet.

Most of the excess accumulation of fat is stored under the skin, especially those areas where it is important in showing a shapely and thin figure, namely the abdomen, hips and arms.

The normal adult has about twenty pounds of fat stored as a reserve upon which to draw under normal conditions such as starvation, or work requiring heavy energy expenditure, or illness. There is enough energy stored in this fat reserve to maintain the essential processes of life for about a month. In the case of malnutrition due to lack of food, or severe illness where food cannot be taken and absorbed, this fat reserve supplies about 90 percent of the energy necessary to still maintain our life.

A most important factor in the regulation of the food we eat and energy storage is the sensation of hunger. Hunger is defined as a sensation of emptiness of the stomach combined with a yearning for food. At more or less regular intervals in the normal person, certain nervous, chemical, an endoctrine (glandular) functions combine to cause an altering series of strong contracting waves to replace the normal slowly-contracting rhythm of the stomach. Such series of waves, or hunger periods, lasts about one-half hour, separated by quiet intervals of one-half to two and a half hours.

If one goes without food too long, discomfort or actual pain may develop (hunger pang). If the person continues to fast, the stomach contractions may continue, but after two or three days the hunger pangs and the general sensation of hunger decreases and may actually disappear altogether.

There are several kinds of hunger . . . fats, carbohydrates (sugars and starches), proteins, salt and water. In the average problem of obesity, excess intake of carbohydrates and fats is the most frequent demanding factor. Some fat we eat is transported directly to the tissues for use as fuel for activity, while part of it is stored in the liver temporarily, where it is changed somewhat for special purposes. The remaining fat is carried directly into the fat deposit areas. So there's your bulky fat, your excess.

Part of the carbohydrates and proteins, consumed in excess, those used for daily body repair and work requirements, is transformed in the liver by a complicated

Here are some hints on what to avoid and look for in your eating. If you are like most people you get 40% of your calories from fat, so eat the foods mostly near the end of the following list:

FOOD	% CALORIES FROM FAT	AMOUNT	CALORIES	GRAMS OF FAT
Whole Milk	48	1 cup	150	8
Ice Cream	48	1 cup	274	14
French Fries	43	10 pieces	137	7
Low Fat Mild	38	1 cup	124	5
Apple Pie	40	1 sm. slice	345	15
Broiled Chicken	25	1 cup	120	3.3
Pizza	25	1 sm. slice	145	4
Low Fat Yogurt	25	1 cup	145	4
Buttermilk	18	1 cup	104	2
Low Fat Cottage Cheese	18	½ cup	103	2
Oatmeal	14	1 cup	130	2
Whole Wheat Bread	13	2 slices	122	1.6
Skim Milk	10	1 cup	93	1
Fresh Apple	9	Medium	82	.8
Tuna Canned in Water	6	4 oz.	144	.9
Cooked Navy Beans	5	½ cup	112	.6
Cooked Brown Rice	5	1 cup	232	1.2
Cooked Split Peas	4	½ cup	115	.5
Banana	2	1 medium	101	.3
Cooked Haddock	2	4 oz.	111	.2
Broiled Potato	.8	1 medium	104	.1
Broccoli	0	1 cup	40	trace
Cooked Lentils	0	1 cup	40	trace
Avocado	91	¼ cup	70	18
Coconut	89	½	190	7
Hot Dog	78	1	170	15
Broiled Sirloin Steak	76	3 oz.	320	27
Cheddar Cheese	71	2 oz.	230	18
Cooked Sliced Bacon	80	2 slices	143	12.5
Canned Cream of Mushroom Soup	68	1 cup	138	10
Poached Egg	68	1	80	6
Tuna Canned in Oil	68	4 oz.	326	23
Cooked Salmon	56	4 oz.	305	19
Milk Chocolate	58	1 oz.	145	9
Chocalate Chip Cookies	53	4 medium	205	12

biochemical process into fat and then stored. Fat is practically the only form in which excessive energy intake is stored, and stored it will be. There is no way of eliminating it other than burning it off.

Stored water normally makes up about 70 percent of the body weight. It may be expected to make up part of the added weight in obesity. In reducing, it is not surprising that one may lose weight after eating food of lower calorie value for several days. Combustion of fat, when one starts utilizing that fat stored in excess, produces water. The metabolism of 100 grams of fat produces 107 grams of water. This water may be only gradually eliminated from the body, and weight decrease may not become apparent until restoration of water balance occurs, (homostasis) in the body.

HERE'S A QUICK CHECK LIST OF WHAT FATS TO AVOID:

Choose lean meat, fish, poultry, dry beans as your protein sources.

Moderate your use of eggs and organ meats such as liver.

Limit intake of butter, cream, hydrogenated margarines, shortenings, coconut oil and palm oil.

Avoid powdered coffee creamers.

Trim excess fat off meat. Skip cream and rich desserts.

Broil, or bake rather than fry foods. Avoid batter and breaded fried foods.

Read the labels and determine the quantity and quality of fats contained in the food.

We all need determination to fight this problem within ourselves. We all find it hard not to be swayed by television commercials and other media presuasions. We all need to be informed surely, but please, not by the hucksters of innuendos and Madison Avenue.

Many experts agree that the typical American diet of over 40 percent calories from fat is too high, and people would benefit by lowering it to at least 10 to 15 percent.

Naturally occurring fats such as those present in whole grains, seeds, nuts, etc. are best. The fats we consume without realizing it are hidden in gravies, dairy products, sauces, pastry, coconut oils and palm oils. Your own health care responsibility must include seeking out the fats that are your own enemies and eliminating them from your diet.

And lastly, any diet that controls weight by restricting calories or carbohydrates certainly is better than the conventional medical way of prescribing amphetamines or other appetite supressants, medications or useless gadgets as are generally available to all of us who yearn to control appetite and lose weight.

SUMMARY THOUGHT!

Remember . . . no fat person has ever broken a longevity record!

Chapter Fifteen
THE BAD WHITE STUFF

"Salt is what makes things taste bad, when it isn't in them."

. . . ANON

By this time I am sure you know that high blood pressure or hypertenstion is a progressive step to artery disease and heart attack. I am almost sure your doctor has told you to stop using salt in your diet. This is almost impossible.

Salt is sodium chloride, and about 40 percent chloride and 60 percent sodium. The important word to watch is "sodium" in food descriptions. You may see wording such as MSG but we should know that it is an additive to enhance flavor and is mono-sodium glutinate. There are sodium nitrate, sodium nitrate, sodium phosphate . . . all food additives, none of which is recommended by any health diet.

This salt or sodium cause high blood pressure and really influences the levels of high blood pressure, or should we say, influences the pressures. Salt is hygroscopic, has the ability to retain water and expand our body's fluid volume. This in turn increases the pressure on the arteries and requires more pumping action.

Diuretics (drugs) such as the commonly used "water pill" are prescribed to reduce excess body fluids and in turn reduce the blood pressure. Many other types of drugs have been used to help this problem, but generally, treatment by diet remains the best I am told, if you know what foods have too much salt and you skip them; if, you know where the sodiums are to skip. Labeling is a loose law.

What makes blood pressure so important is that many scientists believe that many people inherit susceptibility to high blood pressure and high salt diets seem to trigger a heart attack. What's your family history?

If you wish to lower your sodium intake because of the risk, or you have high blood pressure already, you will have a very hard time reducing it even after eliminating salt from your dinner table. You still have no control over the food you eat, regarding salt, unless it is fresh or frozen food.

This is because over 60 percent of the food you buy is processed. So between restaurant foods and meals at home, you have little control over the salt you eat.

To make matters worse, few food processors tell you how much salt or sodium he has in his preparation. The FDA has not gone far enough to label food for salt content. But they are hedging and may someday come up with some token way to give us some idea what to eat and what not to eat, if some pressure is put on them.

Here are some amazing facts you may find difficult to believe as to salt content in the following foods:

Would you believe . . .

Processed Food	**MG Per Serving**
Jello Chocolate Pudding	404
Kellogg's Corn Flakes	260
McDonald's Quarter Pounder	1510
Campbell's Tomato Juice	292
Bacon (is all processed)	302
Heinz Dill Pickles	1137
Breakstone's Low-fat Cottage Cheese	435
Kraft Singles American Cheese	238
Swanson's Fried Chicken	1132
Campbell's Pork and Beans	958
Bumblebee Tuna	628
Wishbone Italian Salad Dressing	315

As you can see, it doesn't matter if its sweet or salty; sour or non-salty in taste; it is processed food. And how do you make processed food inviting to the taste? Just add salt or some sodium product like (MSG) mono sodium glutamate. So the best idea on food consumption is to avoid processed; or if you can, find some processed foods that actually say "No salt added".

When sodium becomes excessive it causes kidney problems and wastes cannot be discharged from the kidney properly causing nutrients to be blocked out. This results in an edema or fluid build up. This condition causes fluid built-up that results in high blood pressure. The importance of sodium/potassium imbalance and the treatment of kidney problems, or hypertension is left to a knowledgable physician so it can be treated in the proper manner for instance the improper use of diuretics for a chemical imbalance.

So here we are again on the dangerous white foods . . . maybe this is what so many dieticians have been trying to tell us for years, eat health foods and raw foods, keep away from processed foods.

AMERICA IS HOOKED ON SUGAR. IT KILLS YOU WITH SWEETNESS.

The average American eats more than 100 pounds of sugar each year. This is too much when we consider, as nutritionists say, you *"get nothing in return but calories."*

Sugar has no nutritional value. White sugar is 100 percent carbohydrate, containing no vitamins or minerals. High sugar consumptions means that there isn't as much room in your diet for better foods; it suppresses your appetite.

To make the sugar matters worse, research has found a relationship between high sugar intake and high blood fat levels, which is suspected of contributing to heart disease.

Cut down on sugar

Eating less sugar can mean reducing the risk of heart disease and diabetes. It can also mean less obesity, dental decay and lowered resistance to infections. Dr. John Cawte, speaking at the first Pan Pacific Conference on drugs and alcohol, said sugar may be the worst substance-abuse threat around. Percapita consumption of sugar and refined wheat flour has increased by 400 percent over the past century. Cawte contends that sugar can become psychologically addictive and that overindulging in processed foods with high sugar content can make people feel dull, lethargic and depressed.

Sugar is the largest ingredient in the American diet. According to the report of the Senate Select Committee on Nutrition and Human Needs, in a report on dieting goals for Americans, it recommends:

Reduce sugar consumption by about 40 percent. According to the report, the most important problem with sugar is that it has no nutritional value, displaces other foods high in micronutrients, and may actually increase the body's need for vitamins such as thiamine, that is necessary to metabolize carbohydrates.

The World Watch Institute, and independent research group, issued a paper called THE TWO FACES OF NUTRITION. Its study showed a per-capita sugar consumption increase of 50 percent since 1950. The study reveals that "health problems" other than tooth decay, painful and expensive as that is, have apparently grown along with the world's sweet tooth. High sugar intake is linked to many studies of diabetes and a host of other diseases.

The study further adds that the affluent American diet, with its increase in fat and sugar consumption and decreases in starch, bulk and fiber has spread, as have a wide variety of diseases such as heart diseases, diabetes, bowel cancer, diverticulosis.

Medical detectives are slowly unraveling the intricate web of inter-connections that link the affluent diet to the various diseases of civilization. Combined with the sedentary lifestyle, high calorie consumption leads to obesity which in turn encourages diabetes, hypertension and coronary heart disease.

The sweet taste boosts appetite even as many dieters switch to sugar-free saccharin products. A recent review by the American Federation for Experimental Biology does not support the opinion that most diabetic foods are a necessity for diabetic diet. Fat fighting dieters have an argument too, that saccharin provides a no-weight addition to the craving for sweetness.

Several studies have found that sugar reduction has been an appetite booster, which may account for the additions and subtractions in daily weight that dieters usually experience.

Dr. Michael Jacobson is a director of the nutrition branch of the Center for Science in the Public Interest (CSPI), a non-profit consumer group in Washington D.C. Dr. Jacobson says, When we consume 20 percent of our calories from sugar, it means we must get all our nutrients from 80 percent of our food. Of course, it is unlikely we are going to get that much nutrition from that food. There are government studies such as the Health and Nutrition Examination Survey that shows a surprisingly high percentage of the population is not consuming the recommended daily allowances (RDA) of nutrients; and one reason is that sugar *is displacing other foods from our diets.*

In as much as sugar intake for the past 50 years has leveled off, it is deceptive becase we are consuming less calories now that we did then, Jacobson says. Sugar is not killing us directly, but rather its pushing good foods, good nutrients, out of our diet, and its hard for us to know what the results will be.

One thing for sure; sugar has become a major factor in American food, that even the diehards who want to eliminate it from their diet find the job of elimination next to impossible. If you avoid every obvious sugar source, such as candy, pastry, cheese, ice cream, and soft drinks completely, you still have a large hidden supply every day in processed foods.

It boils down to the fact that the consumer has developed a sweet tooth craving for sugar and is addicted. That it is harmful and damaging to our society and very hard to refute.

Refined sugar (sucrose), found in processed cereals, contains virtually no nutrients but plenty of calories. It is used to sell more cereals. At the price of sugar today all one needs to do is compare Kellogg's Apple Jacks (57 percent sugar) with Nabiscos Shredded Wheat (1 percent sugar). The TV advertisements rely on sugar's attractiveness for the sales.

To add insult to injury, the remaining ingredients that comprise most cereals are processed; refined grains such as corn, wheat, or rise etc., which are ground, bleached, puffed or toasted using high heat . . . all of which destroy the nutritional value of the cereal. What is left no longer is as nutritionally complete as the whole grain they started with, even when *"enriched"* by the manufacturer.

The next step after creating a cereal almost nutritionally worthless is to enrich it with chemical vitamins and minerals produced in a laboratory, which many believe don't react the same way in the body as natural vitamins and minerals do. Synthetic chemical vitamins are also much cheaper to produce. Sucrose (a fancy word) is refined white table sugar (unless found in nature), the empty calorie type with vitamins and minerals refined out.

HERE ARE SOME SURPRISING FIGURES ON SUGAR PERCENTAGES IN CEREALS FROM A RANDOM LIST:

Commercial Cereal	Percentage of Sugar
Sugar Smacks	61.3
Fruit Pebbles	55.1
Apple Jacks	55.0
Fruit Loops	47.4
Trix	46.6
Frosted Flakes	44.0
Cocoa Krispies	45.9
Captain Crunch	53.5
Alpha Bits	40.3
Sugar Pops	37.7
Sugar Frosted Flakes	29.0
Super Sugar Chex	24.5
All Bran	20.0
100% Bran	18.4
Granola	16.6
40% Bran Flakes	16.2
Life	14.5
Raisin Bran	10.6
Rice Krispies	10.0
Rice Chex	8.5
Grape Nuts	6.6
Wheaties	4.7
Special K	4.4
Product 19	4.1
Puffed Wheat	3.5
Wheat Chex	2.6
Puffed Rice	2.4
Cheerios	2.2
Shredded Wheat	1.3

Heart patients should stay in the low ten cereals for selection. Another way is to make your own cereal as I do. Here's a simple recipe that you can vary to your individual taste or ingredient availability. I call it THE VITALITY CEREAL.

2 parts unflavored soybeans toasted
2 parts sunflower seeds
2 parts whole bran
4-6 parts granola or rolled oats.

1 part wheat germ
add raisins, dates or dried fruit to suit.
Add low fat or skim milk.

It has plenty of calories but it is filling to the stomach thus the appetite is satisfied with less content.

The end does not seem in sight for research and arguments for sugar and its worth to the American diet. We can only hope and look forward to some truth in advertising laws passed in congress that may at least warn the consumer about his annual intake so that he may take such steps as he deems necessary to be healthy and wise.

Some quick tips on your sweet diet,

Cut out jams, jellies, and syrups.
Rely on fresh fruit juice, fresh fruit, not canned or processed.
Cut out all salt, you will still eat hidden amounts.
Avoid salty foods and keep the salt shaker off the dinner table.
Use fresh and frozen vegetables, avoid canned vegetables.
Avoid crackers, pretzels, chips and similar snacks.
Avoid commercial condiments, barbecue, worchester and soy sauces.
Avoid catsup, mustard, relishes and gravy mixes.

Many people have come to believe that bread is the STAFF OF LIFE. This is not true and here is why:

The food industry have very good reasons for providing us with refined flour. It must be economical to market and it must have good "shelf life." In the refinement process oil is removed so it cannot turn the bread rancid. The nutritional life is removed from the wheat berries so the bread cannot be subject ot oxidation. The results is a mass of calories concentrated until they become starch and carbohydrate. This ends up as practically a "dead food," no enzymes, less vitamins and minerals, so they make it difficult for the body to assimilate the white flour in normal metabolism.

So you see the elimination of white flour products such as white bread and rolls, pastry, pie crust, spaghetti, pizza, macaroni, etc., is very necessary.

If you look hard you may find substitutes but you need to read the labels.

I have talked to many people and was quite surprised that they bake their own breads and cakes. My wife and I keep looking and have tried many breads that taste and look good but the ingredients (hydrogenated oils) are contained in all of them, as we are turned off.

We are now eating Arnolds Breads. This somewhat bread specialty company, has many products. Their BRANOLA bread with a variety of ingredients we like very much. They have a whole wheat and oats and bran bread in the variety. Since we get very little bread anymore this taste is very pleasing. There are several brands of crackers in a whole wheat variety also. Here again it is difficult to find all the desirable features talked about in these pages but we keep trying to find the ultimate good tasting healthy eating cracker.

SUMMARY THOUGHT!

IF . . . a majority of people made an effort to cut out the bad white stuff and snack foods; or, if a serious effort were made to prevent cancer, stroke and heart disease, the economy could collapse.

Chapter Sixteen

THE THERAPY OF VITAMINS C AND E

"Middle age is when you begin to exchange your emotions for your symptoms."

... Irwin S, Cobb

From all I can read on the subject, what I have been taught and what I have used, the subject of supplements in our diet, the benefits to our health, the diseases they help treat . . . vitamins C and E are definately the vitamins for your everyday health and the well being of your heart.

Their popularity is not new; they are fast gaining more converts every day. Research has been going on for thirty years on vitamin C, Dr. Linus Pauling is an early and now famous research scientist. Dr. Pauling, Dr. Hans Kugler, Dr. Erwin Stone, Dr. Roger Williams and Dr. Wilfred E. Shute, all have published documented proof in papers of the AMA and other publications. In recent years, this research has led to more favorable publicity for these vitamins, and their use has accellerated at record levels.

The load on the heart is regulated by the oxygen needs of the heart tissues. This demand for oxygen has been found to rise as much as 250 percent in vitamin deficiency. Some variation in response (of each person) is important. Vitamin E acts to slow down tissue oxidation. Vitamin C is important also for it maintains the red blood cells' "oxygen carrying" capacity. If a person is deficient in vitamin C it may cause the blood to lose up to one-half its ability to carry oxygen. The dietary intake of vitamins C and E then can be a matter of life and death. To me, it is a daily intake habit I religiously keep.

Vitamins C and E taken together are instrumental in preventing celluar damage to membranes of the arterial wall and to prevent the formation of plaque. These two vitamins combine to play an active combating part in deactivating cancer-causing chemicals in the body.

The familiar saying "A man is as old as his arteries" implies that old age means developing blood vessel disease. Researchers in molecular chemistry of vitamin C title "The Cement of the Cells" reveals that there is more than a degree of truth in that saying. As the ability of the vessels carrying blood to all parts of the body is extremely important, the prime goal in these studies is to gain improvement over the present condition of the blood vessels.

Vitamin C is a healing vitamin. History shows the action of vitamin C when administered to shock victims and wounded people; improvement has been dramatic and striking. Symptoms resulting from the shortage of vitamin C is a weakening of blood capillaries and the large blood vessels.

The most positive effects of large daily doses, (Dr. Pauling takes 10 *FULL grams* daily) of vitamin C is flavor improvement of food, glandular improvement, lung cell breathing ability, resistance to infection, rapid healing response of wounds, shock recovery, as well as strengthening of all the blood vessels. Vitamin C helps your body manfacture collegen which literally is life strength which builds the walls of our body cells.

Vitamin C saturation, (we do not store it) will give improved daily resistance, better blood, better gums, better blood vessels. Just as vitamin C is important for the repair of damaged tissue, it is equally essential for normal cell regeneration.

Many people know the story of scurvy during the middle ages. There was a lack of fruits and vegetables and soldiers developing hemorrhages of scurvy in their legs. This worked hard on them because of their constant marching. With this reasoning it is quite possible that the regard of physical improvement resulting from increased daily consumption of raw fruits and vegetables may appear in the heart itself, a much harder working muscle than the legs.

Here are some benefits of vitamin C:

- It helps metabolism of the liver and other important body functions.
- In stress situation, vitamin C is exhausted in seconds.

- It combats stress, helps activate vitamin E therapy.
- Helps prevent build-up of cholesterol in plaque, the gooey mess inside the artery walls.
- It is consumed fast in heart attack victims.
- Smokers have low vitamin C levels and need daily doses.
- Lack of vitamin C may cause bleeding, swollen joints and other complications.
- It is found naturally in citrus fruits, tomatoes, raw potatoes and raw green peppers.

The use of vitamin E to reduce oxygen need and therefore increase exercise tolerance has been shown effective in race horses, greyhounds, and in various sports like baseball, hockey, swimming and figure skating.

This effect is because vitamin E is a biological antioxidant. The premature and undesirable oxidation of fats in the blood stream are prevented, and a larger amount of oxygen is reserved for the tissues to take from the blood.

Oxidation, of course, is necessary for normal working of the body, but such a reaction can cause problems also, particularly when it occurs in fats found in the cells membranes and can break the cell open, thereby killing it.

The physical condition in the body, exposure to light, a warm enviroment and exercise are the perfect conditions for oxidation reactions, but because the antioxidants protect the cells from oxidation, the cells remain intact.

Vitamin C and E both can aid measurably in the prevention and have proven to be a help in the relief of heart disease. My exercise program, vitamin supplementation, particularly C and E and chelation therapy certainly helped me to complete relief of leg pain for instance.

The following benefits of vitamin E are as follows:

- Prevents cellular membrane damage from mutagenic and carcigenic elements.
- Regulates fat and protein metabolism.
- Lowers the blood pressure; keeps platelets free flowing.
- Reduces the need for nitroglycerine.
- Keeps the heart younger.
- Prevents some scarring of the heart after an infract and promotes healing.
- Scar tissue wounds and burns heal faster.

- Is a vascodialator; permits nutrients to enter capillaries.
- Helps dissolve blood clots, peripheral vascular artheriosclerosis and insufficiency including intermittent leg pains.
- Involved in synthesis of DNA and RNA.
- Increases blood supply of oxygen by improving "transportation" of oxygen by the blood cells.
- Diabetic and artheriosclerotic retinitis.
- Reduces need for oxygen to the heart, makes the heart more efficient.
- Diabetic and artheriosclerotic early gangerine.
- Increases the blood supply and improves coronary circulation.

Vitamin E is present in fresh whole grain wheat products, many cold-pressed vegetable oils; wheat germ oil, muscle meats, eggs, leafy vegetables, fish, liver and kelp.

It appears that the lack of vitamin E from our daily intake is caused by eating refined white flour, white bread, cereals that are "enriched" with iron. Unsaturated fats, minerals and laxatives exert an antagonistic effect on the utilization of vitamin E.

At home we now eat whole wheat bread and whole wheat crackers or the combination wheat breads that are *naturally enriched.* We try to avoid totally processed foods.

When rabbits were fed no vitamin E in their diets they became paralized. The same thing happens with guina pigs, ducks and even dogs without vitamin E. Under a microscope their muscle fibers showed they were weakened and literally washed out.

As evidence piled up on many discoveries, vitamin E was used in the treatment of fibrosities and other muscular problems. From this successful use and thinking it was but another step to vitamin E's pronouncement as a muscle vitamin. And because the heart is the hardest working muscle in the body, vitamin E was finally classified as a vitamin for the heart. Now today research has confirmed Vitamin E as truly a great heart vitamin.

Those doctors with an education in nutrition and who have studied in this country and abroad and some who have specialized and are experienced in nutrition are the ones capable of making determinations as to the effectiveness of megavitamin therapy and the use of vitamin supplements. Today you can find those professionals who can help in this new improtant scientific field for fighting cancer, arthritis, kidney disease, diabetes, heart disease and other debilitating diseases. The group listings outlined in chapter one would be most helpful to you.

Here are some thoughts I garnered on nutrition and Vitamin C. If you take a fresh orange and squeeze the juice out you should be getting all the vitamin C in that orange, right? Wrong, you are losing almost one-third remaining in the residue. Even if you eat the residue you still lose the nutrition from the orange. This simple fact is true because vitamin C is very sensitive to oxygen. If you blend it in a juicer with some other food you also lose. If its pasturized and packaged in a container you lose.

I have always loved sliced bananas with orange juice for breakfast. I have called it *angel food* since I was a kid. Now I find that Isreal scientists reported in 1978, blended with bananas, oranges lose 75 to 80 percent of vitamin C as it disappears in a reaction of the two fruits.

This is a prime example (and there are many more) or why there are still mystery is nutrition. Why research is still a long way off to all solutions. There are literally thousands of reactions in our bodies and found in the food we eat that is know to scientists and physicians specializing in nutrition. They know many undisclosed complicated reactions that take place in our body. The average person taking food supplements knows nothing except what the manufacturer wants him to know in order to sell the product. This is why I keep repeating why waste money gulping vitamins and minerals when you really do not know or understand if they really benefit **you** individually and directly; not the gullable masses. Remember, there are no rules or guidelines for anyone to follow.

And lastly, nitrates and nitrites alone are not harmful but without vitamin C they form so called cancer causing nitrasomines. Since vitamin C **IS NOT STORED** in the body we need it in our diet every day.

Chapter Seventeen
THE B'S AND THE MINERALS

"When a man dies, he does not just die of the disease he has; he dies of his whole life."

. . . Charles Pierre Peguy

Adding insult to injury, junk foods, soft drinks, candy, pastries, commercial baked goods and hardened cooking fats make up a staggering total of material that is simply unable to build better health and stronger hearts. Therefore the use of these commonly used "non foods" must be curtailed for better heart function.

In review, white flour and white sugar foodstuffs (bread, cake, rolls, buns, waffles, cookies, and ice cream) are all completely without vitamin B needed by the heart, your brain and your nerves.

The use of these foods is harmful because without vitamin B which helps metabolize starch and sugar, they just steal B vitamins from other foods.

Vitamin B-6 found in bananas and raw steak are easily destroyed by heat. This vitamin is essential in metabolism of the many amino acid proteins.

Vitamin B-12 found only in meat and animal products, is essential for normal functioning body cells. The Food and Nutrition Board reports that the body's ability to absorb B-12 may decrease with age.

The trace mineral selenium is also important to our heart action and it enhances the action of vitamin E. It protects human cells from cancer and premature aging. Like iodine, selenium is not found in the soil in many parts of the country consequently our food supply could be deficient. You should check your geographical area to see if selenium is abundant in the soil. The reason is that it has been pointed out in scientific papers that those living in selenium deficient areas of the country are three times more likely to die from heart disease, than those in selenium rich areas.

As research develops selenium benefits are becoming more important such as:

- It normalizes or reduces blood pressure
- Helps protect against plaque formation
- Is important to heart function
- Helps protect cells from cancer, and premature aging.

"Biotin," another B complex vitamin is needed for metabolism of fats, mild deprivation may lead to muscle pains, depression and lack of appetite.

"Niacin" helps circulation, hair growth, cholesterol level reduction, body growth, metabolism and sex hormone growth.

"Choline" helps alcoholism, hardening of the arteries, baldness, constipation, dizziness, ear noises, headaches, high blood pressure and insomnia.

"Vitamin B-1" is a food element that heightens the ability to learn, that recharges your self-esteem and courage. If you have been on a high starch diet B-1 will help melt away nervous tension so common when diets are overloaded with white starches and white sugar and almost devoid in vitamin B-1.

Famine victims of B-1, rich or poor, are generally depressed, always tired, always low in heart tone and vigor. Circulation and emotional problems also develop.

An increased racing heartbeat could mean a lack of B vitamins. The heart races more, as the shortage of B-1 and as the heart beat itself increases. Many people are aware of this functional heart disorder and increasing rate of heart beat. They become short winded, have difficulty in getting their breath on slight exertion, and as a result the heart may become enlarged.

Looking back to the middle of the last century, when grains were first milled, diabetes mellitus has increased over one hundred and twenty percent. Yet it has been repeatedly reported that diabetes was almost unknown among primitive races that only used unmilled whole grain, rich in vitamins of the B Complex family.

For over thirty years, nutritionists have tried to educate the American public into eating whole grain breads. With much advertising support, it is sad to relate only three percent of all the grain breadstuff's sold in this country were made from whole grains.

When you talk to your friends about a switch in diet and away from refined white bread, its a sign of intelligence and knowledge of many health problems. This is wise useage of B complex vitamins contained in whole grain foods.

B-1 is normally stolen from the tissues by consuming white sugar. Synthetic sweetners (used in soft drinks) plus white flour, packaged cereals and generally all sugars such as fructose, dextrose or glucose, all refined and procesed foods, help speed up the dangerous breakdown of tissues. They more or less directly rob the heart and vaso-motor nerves of their thiamine needs (Thiamine cannot be stored in the body).

To burn-up this sugar, the body must steal thiamine from other food sources. This means that if you eat white sugar every day you are almost certain to suffer B-1 deficiency. For those people with heart problems this deficiency could mean grave difficulty.

The number one eating problem for all Americans is the consumption of sugar. Over one hundred pounds consumed a year by each citizen. This is from 60 to 75 pounds more than is needed for our energy and nutritional needs, worst of all, its the wrong kind of sugar.

We injest it in bottled beverages, pastries, commercial baking and the like which are loaded with artificial non-food sugars some of which may be refined. There are about seven spoonfull of sugar in an ordinary soft drink, about a dozen in a piece of ordinary fruit pie.

These deadly overloads of high caloric sweets really get to you to sabotage the body's available nerve-steadying vitamin B. Some time ago a group of scientists at the Mayo Clinic announced that a B complex fraction, nicotinic acid (niacin) assisted in keeping down the amount of cholesterol and related fatty material which tends to increase occlusive artery disease.

The administration of huge doses of niacin, it was reported, lowered the blood cholesterol that had been high in the patients of a large group under study.

While more research may be needed to evaluate the effects of niacin in heart disease, the Mayo study shows strong indications of the importance of certain food elements to health. Unfortunately, such elements are commonly removed from every day foods by refinement. The processing loss includes niacin with its related water-soluble cousin thiamine. All are devoured in the refinement of grains and sugar.

The best way for readers to be properly informed on trace minerals is to have a hair analysis completed so that the report can be thoroughly studied for education purposes by yourself and your nutritional physician.

Some minerals at extremely elevated levels will show some sign of toxicity. Arsenic, lead, cadium, mercury and aluminum will show metabolic effects at very low concentrations, that could produce a disease.

Every mineral taken into the body as food or food supplements should be "chelated" or it is necessary to do it in the body before it is properly utilized. If not chelated or bound, it will stay ionic and in this form, if in excess, will end up forming a stone or calculi.

Science is finding out so many important things about minerals that this writer feels that minerals are better attended for the patients own good, by their nutrition physician.

That the following chart is just a guide for information purposes it does not necessarily advise individuals but rather is a guide for the public.

Choline, Inositol and Phosphorus	Are best given as lecithin, the natural phosphatide derived from soybean, to prevent or reverse enlargement of the liver due to deposition of fat or fatty degeneration. These are the most active of the fatty agents and represent the best therapy for the treatment of high cholesterol in the blood and all the associated diseases alluded to previously. In the form of lecithin, these factors aid in the **utilization of the fat soluble vitamins.**
Minerals and Trace Elements	These are best evaluated by a hair analysis and the following are the most widely reported and the most important:

Calcium	Works in concert with phosphorus, Vitamins A, D, and C. Necessary for normal contractility of heart muscle, nerve transmission and the maintenance of the **delicate acid-alkaline balance.**
Magnesium	Co-enzyme in protein metabolism. Deficiency causes exaggerated response to nerve impulses.
Potassium	Necessary for normal cardiac muscle activity and oxygenation of brain tissue.
Sodium	With K maintains **acid-base balance.** Disturbances produce Adenomas.
Cadmium	Mentioned here because it is a cardiac toxin and when found by hair analysis, should be removed from the body. High doses of Vitamin C and zinc useful.
Cobalt	Essential in production of B-12 in body. Necessary for blood formation.
Copper	Necessary for proper blood formation. Dangerous in excess because it successfully competes with zinc in formation of many enzyme systems especially in the brain, causing schizophrenic disorders.
Iron	Necessary for blood and consequently, oxygenation of all tissues.
Lead	Very common toxic substance, frequently found if looked for. Must be eliminated. Best methods involve high doses of Vitamin C and algin; chelating agents in more severe cases.
Manganese	Necessary in helping zinc compete successfully against copper for enzyme moiety, especially for normal brain enzymes.
Zinc	Necessary for proper brain enzymes, healing processes, insulin formation, normal functioning of prostate gland.

Chromium — Recently discovered by Mertz and shown to be necessary as the glucose tolerance factor, especially in the diabetic.

To better understand the important role of minerals, their vital place in metabolism as well as the danger of some minerals it is suggested that you read the complete paper on hair analysis and its role in mineral detection. See ordering form in rear of book.

SUMMARY THOUGHT!

If I had to choose only one vitamin supplement, to help my heart condition, my top choice would be a total B Complex vitamin.

Chapter Eighteen

STRESS . . . THE BODY / MIND CONNECTION

"All you need to grow fine vigorous grass is a crack in the sidewalk."
. . . Anon.

Every time you excite yourself you can light a fuse on a stick of dynamite that can blow your heart out of circulation. Excitment or stress causes increased reactions in the body and makes demands to all cells of the body. This is like the emotional experiences which make the muscles of the body tense and the mind race. These causes of stress, mean more oxygen is needed and in turn an increase in blood flow.

Stress is the response of the body to any demand put on it. Stress is not simply nervous tension . . . stress occurs in plants and animals as chemical reactions. In humans it is a specific problem which makes us react to seemingly harmful or not harmful circumstances that causes **chemical reaction.**

There are two things we can do to try and overcome stress. Use the right vitamins (B complex and vitamin C) and learn to relax and avoid such stress. We need to do both of these things if we are to avoid heart disease.

The large amounts of sugar most of us eat actually promotes stress as it upsets the delicate balance of blood sugar and insulin. If we cut down on sugar we will have less stress, says Dr. Richard Passwater.

If you smoke it creates stress. Accordingly you need more vitamins A, B complex and E to overcome the consumption of the vitamins that are cancelled by smoking. Just to "keep-up" with stress when smoking you must take in more and more vitamins, or smoke your way to serious problems.

THE HEART 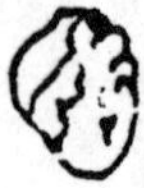	CARDIAC PHOBIAS NEUROCIRCULATORY ASTHENIA NERVOUS OR NEUROTIC HEART HEART DISORDER WITH NEUROTIC SYMPTOMS
THE VASCULAR SYSTEM 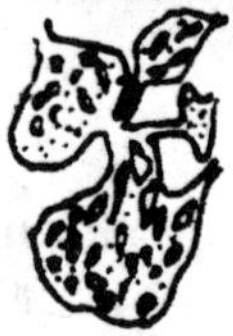	PALENESS EMOTIONAL HYPERTENSION PSYCHIC FACTORS N HYPERTENSION BLUSHING

INFLUENCE OF THE EMOTIONS
Illustrating some results that emotional factors can produce on the heart and on the circulation (vascular system).

Tension occurs when you try too hard to do things that should be done effortlessly or easily. When you are tense, you use energy too freely. In time this process will bankrupt your nerve bank. Your nerves suffer; your arteries tighten, your blood is blocked; and your heart is put under a load. In short, you are ready for a *happening like mine.*

Were it not for the greatest power the body has, the power of self-renewal, we would be finished off in no time at all. Your car or lawn mower can function and wear out but cannot repair itself. Your whole body, including your heart, can repair itself completely, year after year . . . if you furnish the *"right food"* for it.

Norman Cousins in his recent best seller book ANATOMY OF AN ILLNESS and his story of incurable disease, says the last place you should be is in a hospital when you are sick, that hospital's are a very stressful environment. Cousins also says in his book that ten minutes of solid belly laughter would give him two hours of pain-free sleep.

The implications here of Cousins and other research and practicing scientists are that our habits, stressful situations, our nervous system are all inter related.

Today, various metaphysical, therapeutic touch, foot reflexology, biofeedback, psychobiology, autogenic training, or other healing methods, are in use. All these efforts are being administered on hopeless cases of various diseases, all with various degrees of success.

Here are some chosen words from a former surgeon turned physchiatrist. With well rounded experience Dr. Wallace Ellerbroek of Metro State Hospital in Norwalk, California calls stress a positive effect. He says depression is behind all mental and physical disorders. If you think all sorts of screwy things you get sick. This is not an incident that happens to you, but something you do to yourself. For instance he says one does not have cancer, but rather one is cancering.

Dr. Ellerbroek says it depends on our own inward thinking, as fantasy of how things ought to be does not match the fantasy of how things are now, that we get into trouble. And thinking that you can do something about it makes you angry, and thinking that you can't do anything about it makes you distressed and frustrated. These are states of responsibility for all of us to ponder, intimates the doctor, as the cause of disease.

Dr. Kennith Pelletier has said that 1971 started this professional change in thinking, mostly caused the rapid growth of heart disease and the impact made on professionals and the public alike. Type A behavior has been classified by many and he says it is being short tempered, impatient, agressive, always ready to fight a deadline and includes any person, even a child, a car in traffic that refuses to yield, a secretary problem or a pressing boss. Pelletier says that if you get frustrated over minor things you could give yourself a heart attack.

Scientist like Pelletier can boil down the problem of stress to six factors that you can make a fairly accurate prediction on just what diseases a person is likely to get. That is a big mouthful on predictability and will be covered in the chapter on prevention. These include physical activity, biological factors, genetic and nutritional factors as well as physicological profiles.

There are other factors relating to causes of stress.

Psychiatrist Dr. Barbara Betz of Southern California Permanente Medical Group in Los Angeles offered her views taken from such studies. Dr. Betz speaks of temperment given to us at birth that is an inborn disposition that may be handed down from a parent. She said that there is sort of learned behavior resulting from everything that has happened to you, its called personality. Nurses in new born nurseries know that babies are not all alike; from the moment they are born they can see the calm smiley ones, the shy ones and the little stinkers. Betz reminds us that temperment does not have to do with cognative skills but with various traits such as vivacity or calmness; things that are recognized in the dog breeding world.

I read somewhere that disease is a process of running yourself down or coming apart; and health is a process of energizing and coming together. That when the body, mind and spirit are NOT in harmony we become sick and when everything seems just fine we are well.

The high cost and ineffectiveness of present-day medicine has turned many people off. Consequently more and more doctors are gradually learning to be involved in the new exciting field such as holistic medicine.

Pelletier says we were sort of switched off when sulfa drugs and infectious disorders like polio were conquered. What should have happended was that we were supposed to live longer and health lives. We did *not* have healthier lives. Instead there was an increase in non-infectious and non-specific stress related disorders like ulcers. These ulcers are just part of what Pelletier claims represents 50 to 80 percent of all disorders in the United States caused at least in part by stress.

We need to examine all the literature in this field and in doing so come to the conclusion that virtually all states of disease, all states of our health are at least in some degree psychosomatic. This includes heart disease, cancer, respiratory disease and arthritis even inflammatory virus disorders are stress related.

Many readers are going to dispute the findings of the experts. They are going to use examples to point out their own rebutted thinking. Their friends who lived long lives while dissipating to the highest level of smoking and/or drinking. Or, why does one two-pack-a-day smoker get lung cancer and another just as heavy a smoker live a healthy happy life? Or, why a heart bypass patient who also had chelation therapy afterwards, also continue smoking and not be affected during his continued life span.

Why, in this environment conscious world, almost everything we breath, drink or eat is thought to be carcinogenic, yet nearly all of us don't get cancer? There are many arguments that can be made for most every condition in this world. But, in view of both sides of this particular argument, at least we get the message loud and clear, and enought to lead us to more research already under way. To find the "connection" between the spirit and the flesh; between a healthy body and a healthy mind.

The bottom line is quite simple if we think about it. You are healthy when you are yourself. Do anything that gives you a sense of joy and enthusiasm.

I am sure you are convinced there is a connection between the body and the mind and how the mind affects the body and how the body affects the mind and how the environment works on both. The body/mind connection adds up to a new respect for an ancient dictum, *NATURE HEALS, NOT THE PHYSICIAN.*

As we have discussed, there is a new movement today of more-or-less a grass roots variety. We have mentioned holistic medicine, orthomolecular therapy, megavitamin therapy, and holistic health. In this new movement taking place we see examples of the art in healing cancer by the use of megavitamins. We see the healing power of prayer, the Christian belief, transdendental meditation, yoga, hypnotism, autogenic training, and other healing processes. These processes work, each of its own degree.

The question is do they work by reducing stress, or are there active forces that promote good health? Biofeedback machines have shown we can use mental control over inner processes. Physicists keep coming up with intriging evidence about our light force. We are learning that innate therapy such as these are more miraculous than any single purpose drug.

Evidently when functioning, this force triggers our immunization system to ward off the viruses we all live with. It gives us that unknown resistance to cope emotionally, in this stressful world.

How to capture this process and keep it going for us is where all hope lies. And while we seem limited in results from these healing arts, we hear people on TV enthusing about new vigor and successes, the tabloids discussing "miracle healing." The subject has made Playboy Magazine April 1981 right behind the centerfold. Author Don Black takes a look at this new movement. Where there is smoke there is fire could be true as we look into the near future.

This is a mixed picture that is drawing unlikely practicioners, from a few members of the AMA to a growing breed of *"alternate health givers."* The talk of what makes us tick, get sick, stay well, and those ideas worry the AMA old guard.

This new approach is an invitation to health that conjures up hope as well as consumer caution. But you are reminded to keep away from the formerly vauge "mind over matter" notions we hear ocassionally. Rather it should be saying to you that mind and emotions are expressing illness in our matter (body).

Dr. Hans Selye put the word "stress" in our medical language. Everyone reading a popular magazine knew about those *bad old tensions.* The message as recognized is, *unrelieved anxieties can be a killjoy or eventually a killer.*

The close connection between emotions and the body is nowhere so evident as in the circulatory system. The story of the broken heart, the rejected lover, of the sweetheart given up, of betrayed women or the mother that a lost a child, and the heart which suddenly stops beating with joy, upon receiving unexpected news of a loss of a beloved one . . . all such stories have been told for countless years.

In this connection we must emphasize that the "painful heart" is an expression and a consequence of some emotional disturbance of dissatisfaction, and fear, worry and frustration.

There's no denying that on the basis of long-standing psychic cardiac disturbances, organic disease may develop and pre-existing alteration may, under an emotional upset, turn into serious physical problems. Such emotional upsets again are dangerous to heart patients.

There's a new book this year published by Bobbs-Merrill called TOTAL RELAXATION by Frederick P. Lenz. The author is a student of Eastern medication techniques. He scoff's at the popular versions of Transcendental Meditation. He says they are not for relaxation as much as they are for attaining altered states of conciousness, which is a lifetime commitment. He says his book promises to change your life if you take it seriously, as indeed, most so-called holistic programs can do if they are followed scrupulously.

Here Lenz is most helpful with a list of stress reducers:

- DRIVING YOUR CAR. Don't get into an agrument with a passenger especially one in the back seat. On a three-lane highway, don't drive in the right lane (entering and exiting traffic is stressful.) Avoid loud music.
- JOB HUNTING. Take an extra pair of shoes with you; one for interviews, the other for walking between interviews.
- BOREDOM. Watch public television instead of the same old shows or soap operas. If house work is boring have someone else do it for you.

Lenz rightfully singles out television viewing for a good part of his criticism. He says that television is the greatest cause of tension and fatigue in the home. That as we waste hours in front of it we are subjecting our conciousness to a almost contineous mish-mash of useless stimuli that results in a tired feeling of frustration, that unfullfilled feeling at the end of the evening. He suggests that we observe the commercials and how they are designed to subliminally brainwash us. It we analyze them we will note all types of false expectations that are being forced on us. Be aware of the process so that you will not be affected.

Too many Americans try to manage stress by taking dangerous tranquilizers. This crutch only treats symptoms, not the causes, and may impair the ability to reason over the long term. Experts recommend learning how to relax and find a combination of stress-management techniques that can work for you.

Heart attack victims score very high on Type A rating scales. Myer Friedman the Author and Ray H. Rosenman, published in 1974 (Alfred A. Knoph), popularized the concept so many professionals have investigated thoroughly. TYPE A BEHAVIOR AND YOUR HEART allows you to rate yourself with a check list of behavior patterns. Heres a sampling:

- Squeezing too many activities into too little time.
- Attempting to hasten the speech of others.

- Attempting to always be on time.
- Trying to do two things at once.
- Talking with your hands.
- Difficulty sitting still and doing nothing.
- Explosive speech patterns, profanity, loud talk.
- Irritation while waiting in line.

If you have had a heart attack already you should know about these health habits that cause problems. If you have symptoms you had better pay attention carefully to this list of bad habits.

After being saved from death at Little Big Horn . . . Little Big Man realizes he isn't dead and said, "Once you should have died and didn't, you ain't never the same."

To live each day as if it were your last may be good advice, but suppose you say, "I live each as if I am going to live to be a thousand years old; I have that great feeling, just to be alive! That's what you may need to eliminate stress.

SUMMARY THOUGHT!

There are about 750,000 Americans walking around like Zombies, taking Valium and other tranquilizers regularly. About half of them can look forward to more of the same and irreversable stress conditions with much more serious problems. They have accomplished little or nothing in the process. They are not cured or helped. They have just placed their minds on an irremovable crutch, they still have the condition.

Chapter Nineteen

HOW OLD IS OLD?

"Real joy comes not from ease and riches, or from the praise of men, but from doing something worthwhile."

. . . Sir Wilfred Grenfell

I don't know---you don't know---how old is "OLD"? Most people say you are only as old as you feel. In today's hustle and bustle world, you could have a sixty-year old heart and a forty-year-old body. A person could start on the road to decline at thirty-five or forty years of age, yet his mother may be witty, gay and active at seventy-five years of age. *Why do we want to live longer?* It should be a question of *"Why do you want to die sooner?"*

Extended long life doesn't seem to be of interest to many older people I have talked to on the subject and tried to pep-up. Possibly they are mentally down on their own health problems that prompts disinterest. Many believe as they grow older their present health problems will increase to the "lost hope" stage. Some believe they are already in this stage.

This is psychological aging, as we become aware of our dimishing capacity. Then to make it worse, losing optimism for the future, by short-sighted foolish thinking.

Still, I believe that as older people are showing that they actually can reverse their aging process or at least slow it down, they will not only change their thinking but they will start changing their habits and lifestyles. Many older people are already setting good examples.

In fact, its so easy to do that more and more older people are now entering this "changed phase" leaving behind the debilitating effects of sedentary television living. A look at the chart holds a key as projected age extensions rapidly rise.

Heart efficiency and the circulating system can be better understood if we learn the mechanism by which the body and its arteries, blood and the heart are renewed and strengthened.

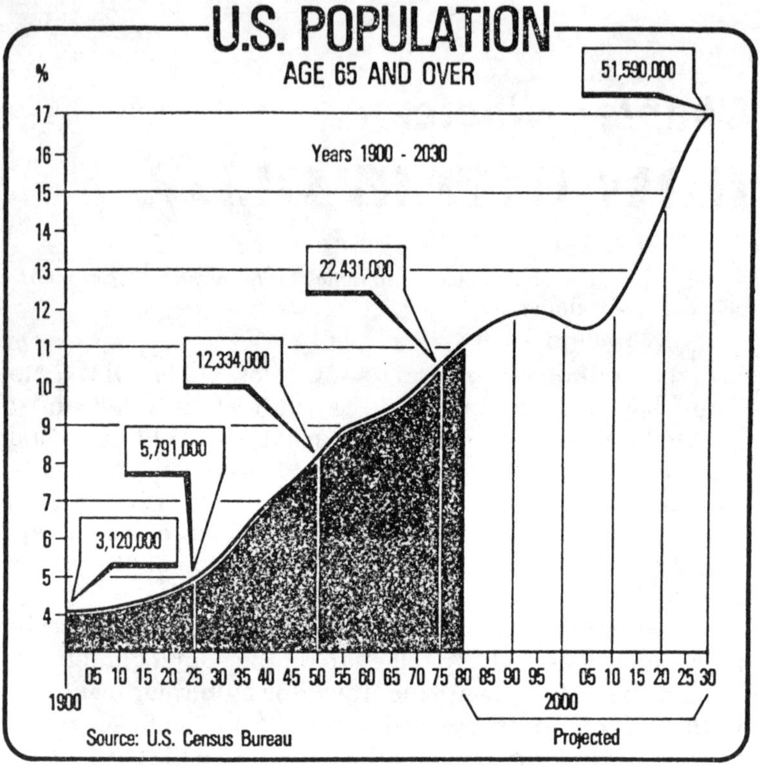

AGE GAUGE — Chart shows the percentage of the American population 65 and older from 1900 to 1975, with predictions for 1980 to 2030.

Within the body, Mother Nature has placed a red blood cell renewal clock that completes its cycle about every thirty days. (women have similar menstrual cycles) The Atomic Energy Commission said long ago that the body registers a renewal of 89 percent of the body each year.

The speed of life in its long length or shortness, makes every living thing timed like a "clock"; some live faster than others and so life burns faster. A dog's life is seven times faster than a human life. The tiny hummingbird has to eat almost continuously and lives about 100 times as fast as an elephant; to support the humming bird's small body, it burns its food up as fast as it eats it.

All scientists view it in various years but I have read that they believe the biologic "clock of life" for humans is wound up to last about 125 years. The Bible confirms this in

Genesis 6:3, "and his days shall be a hundred and twenty years."

There is scientific theory for this extension of life theory. Now today, new breakthroughs are being made in this field of aging. The 125 years limit is being pushed upward. "I am convinced that we are on the verge of major advances in what we know about the biomedical mechanisms of aging," declared Senator Alan Cranston (D. Calif.) who is monitoring progress being made. "In fact, the work being done today is so phenominal that," the Senator flatly declares, "we might be able to stretch the healthy middle years of life into the 70s or 80s or beyond."

Senator Cranston, a member of the Senate Health and Scientific Research Subcommittee, has met with many of the top experts on aging and says he knows of amazing developments. "What I have heard from these experts is astonishing to laymen." Cranston explained.

Many leading researchers also agree with his knowledge and enthusiasm. Dr. William Regelson, professor of medicine at the Medical College of Virginia in Richmond, agrees and declares it is going to hit us so fast that our heads will spin in disbelief. The mere mention of middle age being 70 to 80 years appears to be conservative and is going to happen for sure, said the doctor.

The work with laboratory animals over the years has established full support for the expectations of these researchers. For instance Dr. Denham Harman, a University of Nebraska biochemist, has found substantial evidence that aging is caused by *FREE RADICALS;* parts of molecules that have broken loose in the body and cause damage to cells. By giving certain chemicals to mice, Dr. Harman has been able to slow down the formation of free radicals in their bodies.

Dr. Harman has said to significantly increase the life span of mice as much as 20 percent and in one case up to 44 percent. This is very significant when we realize this life span increase in the lowly mice is like increasing mans life span by about 10 years. It has been proven that mice and man compliment the same comparable method of study.

You will be hearing and reading a great deal about "free radicals" and their effect on the aging process, it appears here lies some answers to slow down premature aging.

Researcher Richard Hochschild at the University of

California at Irvine, is working on a way to repair damage to a cell that has been attached by a free redical. They are membrane stabilizers, a compound that will repair the cell membrane and help strengthen it against any future damage. Such mice that received the compound had their life span increased from 20 to 40 percent above normal, the researcher stated.

Dr. Regelson believes we will soon be shown proof that senility is reversable, that what we are talking about is the maintenance of the youthful state. (Chelation therapy has helped senility) Regelson says this is not pie in the sky talk and his belief and enthusiasm seem to make his work very exciting. Since this speculation on life span naturally involves the heart, we should realize that this is where our own responsibility lies and action starts.

Why does the heart of an elephant weaken at about 50 years and the small carp can carry on for as long as 100 years? We have found that crocodiles lay eggs that are fertile 200 years later, while a tiger's heart may weaken before 20 years. Blood circulation, cardiac strength we have learned are basic to this fact but we are near to gaining all the details for summary information.

Its easy to see eye changes in people after 40 years of age, and more changes occur later on. On the mental side, we see people with high intelligence growing more intelligent as the years go on, while lower intelligent people lose vocabulary and their ability to learn new things. We now know there is a vast difference in biological aging and chronological aging.

With intelligent appreciation and application of the known facts, premature old age may be held off for many years. We are seeing it applied in many ways in preventive medicine, through nutrition, holistic techniques and the "back to basics" thinking of the early years of this century.

If you are skeptical, or easily discouraged, go to the public library and find out all these facts. If you are set in your ways, there are well validated records as well as up-to-date reporting. Possibly such proof will help motivate you to start thinking young. So keep an open mind as we unravel this need for a new way of life.

I recently sat alongside of and talked at length to a patient taking chelation treatments. He is 87 years of age. What was wrong with him you ask? Old age disease? No, Nothing much was wrong with him. Walter Whitt vows to live to be 100 years of age. He had a pain in his hip and was trying to get rid of it with DMSO therapy and decided to take ten chelation treatments also as a preventive measure.

The man is a bundle of vitality; his color is excellent and you would guess his age at about 60 years. He swims daily, watches his diet, takes food supplements and is the life of activity (here lies the key) among those persons receiving chelation treatment. Looking at this man, I marvel; seeing him up close, I am mystified; talking to him I am convinced that he will easily reach his goal of 100 years. While writing and learning what I have been researching, I am convinced he will exceed that goal by many years.

Fighting for a victory against old age is real warfare. You are lost if you adopt an easy going attitude concerning it or neglect a single weapon against it. Every mouthful of the wrong food, and every weak muscle or laziness helps to conquer you.

Its time we all accept that the passing years have, by themselves, little effect on our body. Only when a man or woman lives wrongly does looking older become a reality as the years pass. Senility and degenerative old age are signs that the human body has adapted itself to bad foods, a soft life, and bad surroundings. There's nothing but gradual deterioration left and the usual catastropic ailments.

This is where I found chelation therapy treatments can get you started on the road back, and preventive medicine as outlined here can prolong lives, and reverse the aging process for many beneficial years.

The main point I could make is that anything that damages your body will also age it. Chemistry and the mind combine in a wonderful partnership in a healthy body that moves the spirit. More than any creation, the human cells bear witness to Almighty God as Creator. These are the materials you work with in your switch over to biologic, heart-toning, heart strengthening living and eating.

A well known writer about the effects of negative emotions on health is James J. Lynch Ph.D. a professor at the University of Maryland School of Medicine and author of THE BROKEN HEART: THE MEDICAL CONSEQUENCES OF LONLINESS. (Basic Books 77). Dr. Lynch says we live in a mechanistic society and look into the physical area for causes of sickness, such as an infectious disease. In doing so we fail to see the social and phychological factors in health and longevity. Dr. Lynch said that people need to relate to one another as well as love one another which is the basic effect on health.

Then there is researcher Michael K. Miller Ph.D. a sociologist at the University of Arkansas at Fayetteveiie who talks about our medical system being at fault. That it is treatment after the fact, we should be dealing with up front rather than emphasize critical intervention. The good doctor mentions the serious consequences produced from too much surgery and the medical error involved. Dr. Lynch says he don't consider it health care since lifestyle is the prime factor in why we are unhealthy. Of course he emphasizes what have been reading here: low fat diet, no smoking, exercise, reducing weight so we can add 7 to 11 years to a persons lifetime.

PREVENTION IS THE KEY. YOU MUST TAKE CARE OF YOURSELF AND BE IN CONTROL OF YOUR OWN HEALTH.

Statistics show that life expectancy has increased more than 50 percent during the first three-quarters of this century. You can live well past the 70-80 range as the result of new medical research, active lifestyles, and renewed eating habits. So why spoil your chances for added life expectancy during the last fifth of this century.

By now you should be convinced that premature old age, infirm bodies, weak or clogged arteries, and low body tone or sickness does not "just happen." The right sort of living will usually result in improved health, because we were never intended to be sick in the first place.

By the very same power by which Mother Nature closes a cut or heals a wound, builds a new bridge over broken bones or digests food, she can raise your heart tone, improve your arteries and increase blood circulation. Really, your age has little to do with it. How you eat, how you use your muscles, how full a life you live intelligently, has everything to do with it.

Dr. Garry F. Gordon, in an interview in Ft. Lauderdale, Florida prior to a "Slowing the Aging Process Seminar" stated, "Chelation therapy holds the possibility that angina pain can be wiped out eventually. It will cancel the need for up to 80 percent of bypass operations and at one-tenth the cost."

As we discuss aging and chelation therapy, keep in mind that the entire program of prevention is intended to reverse the biological process of aging. Biological aging can be slowed down to permit you a younger and healthier chronological aging.

The 1980s already indicate more research, more answers that we have been seeking and many breakthroughs are very near. Don't miss it. Its the only life you will ever have.

"WE ARE AS OLD AS OUR ARTERIES" . . . WILLIAM OSLER, M.D. 1894

SUMMARY THOUGHT!

EXPERTS' RECIPE FOR A LONG HAPPY LIFE

Instead of television, try painting, bowling, needlepoint, dressmaking, gardening, or other activities that excite your mind and body. No matter your physical or financial status, join church, political or other activities. The rocking chair is not the successful formula. Hope and despair have no room in a solidarity movement of physical or social activity.

Chapter Twenty

BODY MOTION FOR HEALTH

"Practice does not make perfect, perfect practice makes perfect."
. . . Vince Lombardi

Body motion seems like a better word than exercise, particularly when we are talking to victims of heart disease and stroke and the debilitating effects of sedentary life. Exercise is just body motion in any form at all, from moving your fingers to making a fist; from walking or jogging to calesthenics. Since the body was meant to be used well and hard, the more movement it gets, the healthier it becomes. Why?

First, the body has to be fed with food and energy; if it is not fed it will slowly die; if it is not fed the proper foods, cells will die off, unneeded fats will accumulate, and without the energy and activity to *"burn off"* the excess fat, we are in trouble. The maintenance and health of the body depends on movement to keep circulation up, to keep oxygen and blood flowing freely, to keep the muscle tissue up to par, by *activity.* Too little activity makes us sluggish, and causes your vital organs to *slowly waste away.*

When we reach forty years of age and up, it is necessary that we all exercise *more, not less,* as so many keep telling themselves. Exercise is medicine that stimulates the body so we can synthesize the high-density lipo-proteins (HDL) (fats); these are fats that are hard to break-up or dissolve. Doctors look at these HDL to determine risk factors of build-up of plaque and cholesterol in heart disease. Sedentary life goes hand in hand with overweight. All clues to inactivity.

Most important, body motion and activity leaves us with a feeling of well-being and alertness for long periods after the activity is over. Many times you are tired at first, then quickly the tiredness leaves, resulting in that feeling of stimulation and satisfaction. Ask any regular practicing exerciser.

The American Cancer Society has a study that shows the death rate of men 45 to 65 who exercise regularly is *four times lower* than those men who do not exercise.

Someone said, "An ounce of exercise is worth a pound of prevention." Often the difference between life and death lies in the amount of collateral circulation to the heart that has been developed after a heart attack. It is only through exercise that the heart gains such activity and such an *auxiliary* blood and oxygen supply.

Inactivity has been shown to cause an increase in cardiovascular and ventilatory demands, for any given quantity of exercise . . . this is a state referred to as *"deconditioning."*

There is plenty of publicity and discussions going on now about jogging and it seems to have started a craze. While basically they jog for health, I believe most people are motivated by the high cost of getting sick.

I really do not think that jogging is necessary as a health measure, particularly the incessant need for unlimited endurance. But I can emphasize most assuredly that if we all walked more, we would all have many less problems.

Since the automobile age, we have become the most urban people in the world. Our lives are insulated from air, the ground, the light, and even from each other. The car, air-conditioner, and buildings all form barriers. And yet if we are aware, sensible, and wise, we must get back in touch with the elements, with nature itself. In this regard, perhaps the rising price of gasoline may be a blessing.

We must put our feet on the ground every day automatically . . . so we can touch what is best in this creation and exercise our minds and senses in a vital way, to appreciate the world around us.

If walking were encouraged more for all of us, there would emerge a better closer-knit people and a healthier overall climate with less pain and agony. Think what would happen if everyone walked more and used their cars only 50 percent less. We used to do it, before the automobile age. There was less sickness then, too.

We would be able to make many more friends by striking up more conversations; have better communications between ourselves and with others. While walking, we see more around us, to feel these elements and get to appreciate nature more, allow for friendly curiosity and sociability, to sense the meaning of all of God's creation all this as we walk along.

Isn't this better than exhausting and deteriorating driving that leads to a blank mind or stress or high blood pressure? I know for a fact that walking makes the blood circulate better and the imagination to bubble. I get most of my ideas and am able to think more clearly and rationally while I am walking in the early morning.

In recent studies, doctors have observed that women who walk around in early labor have easier births than those who allow themselves to be treated as hospital cases.

The benefits of walking can produce fantastic results. We have conditioning for better healthy bodies, and savings from health care expense; both can be substantial in this rising battle with inflation. Surely the reason we see much more activity today.

As we are forced to pay more and more for the real costs of consuming energy the family car will become less attractive. We had better start getting used to walking. People are thinking about short-cuts to high medical bills now. The answer lies in more walking and less, costly car use.

On this basis alone, we should encourage others to walk with us and develop habits and attitudes together and develop a partner-encourager, the habit-forming attitude of many walkers evergrowing into still more walkers. In return we have an achievement that will affect our lives and save more energy than we can hardly believe possible.

In turn, we will develop good interesting activities, as well as a good healthy life. The troubles and coldness of driving a car will be alleviated as we recognize human beings with two legs with the ability to stride, to stroll, or to saunter our way to health.

When I lived in Ohio eight years ago, I exercised in a public school gym winter and summer for at least one hour, three mornings a week.

I needed it, and knew it, for every time I got out of my car after a rather long drive I was stiff, half bent over, and numb in the rump. That's all a traveling salesman really does each day you know, drive and drive. Between stops you would walk about 50 yards and drive some more, all day long. You eat in between, go home and relax and eat again; then go to bed, only to start the same boring routine over again the next day.

We played three-or-four-man, one-basketball, and loosened up into shape for the 7:10 a.m. program. For a solid 20 minutes we did a series of routine calesthenics and then went home. Really, I felt great all the time; it was good medicine and it helped me constantly on my job. In fact, I firmly believe it attributed to the recovery from my heart attack.

When we moved to Florida it was too hot to play golf, too hot to exercise, or I was just too lazy. Many of us know about this lazy condition as we grow older and do little or no exercise, the greatest of which is turning on the television. So here I was back again traveling long distances and driving myself into the same old routine. So what happens? "My happening" . . . a heart attack.

Let me briefly describe my exercise program after and during convalescence and up to the present date. All I could do at the start, upon returning home from the hospital, was leisurely slow walking for a short distance. This increased gradually until finally I was up to about one and one-half miles in about eight weeks. Then brisk walking started after about a dozen chelation treatments. This increased to 45 minutes and is now one hour. I stop at one hour, but do it daily. I am tired, soaking wet with perspiration, but very soon after feel fine, rested, and refreshed again.

During these progressively increasing distances, I knew when to extend myself and by how much by the pain in my left arm. As the number of chelation treatments increased, the walking also increased and the pain in my arm lessened. The more chelation treatments, the less pain in my arm until finally the pain was gone. Incidentally, the pain in the arm was part of the previous angina pains. It usually started in the chest and then went to the arm, before I needed a nitroglycerine pill. I have not taken a nitro tablet since the chelation treatments started. Long before that I abandoned the nitro ointment patch that had to be stuck on my skin three times a day.

Exercise stimulates the bones and helps bone maintenance by standing and walking, and protects bones from wasting away. Why do hospitals get you out of bed as soon as possible after an operation? To stimulate by exercise, of course.

If you work behind a desk, you know the benefit of going for a drink or to the john, or for a coffee break. But if this is your work and habit alone, chances are you are worse off by far than, say, the active factory worker or mailman.

If you eat too much, or eat the wrong foods, chances are that this problem can be mostly overcome by physically active work to burn off calories and to reduce chances of a heart attack.

Some say if you exercise you tend to eat more. This is not true as studies have shown that exercise dulls your appetite right before meals. I try to walk or exercise **before** meals. So trade in your rocking chair for a pair of comfortable walking shoes and get going. Don't believe that old-time culture we learned, to *expect* to slow down and degenerate as we grow older.

I asked my doctor about my infarct (scar on the heart) where the heart attack affected it and that spot died. He said the dead spot on my heart was the reason for the exercise, to stimulate the area around the infarct so it will grow new blood vessels (collaterals) to supplement the damaged ones, and that is just what Mother Nature does for you by exercise.

To be cured of the overweight problem you need exercise and diet. That **extra weight taxes your heart** to pump more blood through the extra fat area where you naturally have built up additional blood vessels.

Other than walking, I supplement calesthenics with gardening and lawn care. I also raise cuttings to plants and make my own compost. I occasionally jog a bit but I don't need to . . . I feel great.

I have called on thousands of retired people, the great majority of them are on many different pills for every ailment imaginable. I was amazed to see his and her piles of various drugs in virtually every home of retirees. Unfortunately most of these people just sit around and watch television and waste away ever so slowly from inactivity and the effects of the drugs. The worse off these people are health-wise, the less they do in the way of exercise. Naturally they don't feel well, so they take it easy, too easy. They fall into a rut or slump and usually stay there, and they won't feel any better unless they get their bodies out of that chair and back into shape. The pills put them on a *"holding pattern";* they do some good but they don't affect the cure. They just exist. Possibly they have been listening to **their doctor who tells them to take it easy**. So they wait until something happens, putting in the time wasting slowly away. And they wait and finally that something else . . . ?

I have asked several doctors about these people. They are well known to the new breed of medical professional. They tell me that there is nothing that can be done to motivate them, usually. They are too set in their ways and as one said they are "too pooped to pop." This is a sad commentary in such a knowledgable world. This is the control of our lives I speak about when referring to the AMA.

For older folks, walking only brief distances and build up distances as you start to feel better from it; never over tire yourself but try and extend yourself each time just a little more. But remember, it must be done regularly. If you get leg cramps, stop walking till the pain ceases. Tell your doctor about the pain. Another idea for the older folks to start. Take exercise before you get out of bed. Move your toes, feet, hands and arms, stretch and do exercises lying down. Try the bicycle act while in bed or on the floor.

While walking tones the body and mind, the key benefits are:

• *RELIEVES DEPRESSION.* There are all sorts of theories on this, but basically there are chemicals released as neurotransmitters or pain killers.

• *REDUCES ANXIETY.* Walking dissipates anxious energy that is not being used. Using energy makes us less tense.

• *AIDS IN BUILD-UP OF ESTEEM.* Brisk walks stop people from accepting the idea that their bodies are deteriorating. It shows them they can CHOOSE to be healthy.

• *CREATES A SENSE OF EXHILERATION.* Instead of being tired out, these people find they have MORE energy to get to work and they find they are less aggressive in their life at home. In short there is more energy because they have improved their circulation, there is more oxygen in the body. Exercise is a general toner of the body and the mind, which really is our whole individual system.

I read an article about Bonnie Pruden, the well known, and most likely the original exercise girl on television. She is now 63 years of age. She says older folks can get in shape in six to eight weeks. Why? Because we are born before the push-buttom age. We walked to school, ran to the store for our mothers, and pushed lawnmowers. We did heavy housework without the use of electrical appliances and had regular eating and sleeping habits. She too says you needn't get out of bed to exercise, and that the human body, unlike the machine, *IMPROVES WITH AGE.*

One of the most important and vital movements for the older person has to do with breathing . . . slow deep breathing. Good for smokers and non-smokers. No matter your age, it should be done daily. One way is by standing and using the arms in a raising motion while inhaling,; holding the position momentarily, then slowly lowering the arms to a rest position while exhaling.

Done about ten times a day, it puts your lungs in shape by giving them more capacity for air, keeps the lungs "toned up" so they are able to provide a full supply of oxygen to the blood, heart, and body.

I read about a nutritionist who was discussing proteins. He said that protein's main job is to help rebuild tired muscles; that proteins are not the primary or secondary source of energy. For physical work, proteins won't make you stronger; only exercise will make you stronger. Too much protein turns to fat or is excreted . . . it is rather easy to eat too much protein. More importantly, exercise burns up calories, and is so easy to do when it concerns your health.

Exercise is needed not only for good health, but it is an inexpensive pasttime. It can turn the boredom of inactivity into a refreshing living experience.

It is self-defeating to be ailing, lying around doing nothing, in many cases just wasting away. This is the time you can use to defeat "father time." The time to exert effort in some form of activity regularly, each day. It will pep you up and help you laugh at the world again; it will help you back to health by increased activity.

For some readers, there was a time you probably used to enjoy exercise, but now you feel that sit-ups or other exercise is just a little too strenuous for you to handle at your age. You are wrong because you can start building up the exercise slowly, little by little. Look around you, there are others older than you keeping active and happy. Its time to give yourself a pep talk and move it, move anything but move it. Again, walking is the one exercise where you cannot lose anything but time. But walk only brief distances to start, and never overtire yourself. Legs cramps could occur but as you stop and rest remember it is a sign of poor circulation and you need to see your doctor.

And lastly, even a rocking chair is good exercise if it is used as an exercise tool. It brings into use toes, feet, legs, and finger muscles by gripping the chair firmly and releasing them in some sort of unison. This may even promote a relaxing mood.

But please, do not use your easy chair as a crutch. Crutches are hard to get rid of. Get up and walk, keep away from that easy chair in front of the television. You'll be glad you did. Make tomorrow the body motion way to the rest of your great life.

SUMMARY THOUGHT!

If your dog is fat, you are not getting enough exercise.

Chapter Twenty-One

WATER THE BODY SOLVENT?

"Water taken in moderation, cannot hurt anyone."
. . . Mark Twain

Most of us remember when people could safely drink their own tap water and even from lakes and streams. Today, everyone knows this is no longer true. Even our own tap water is badly polluted and contaiminated and people have long since given up drinking from streams and lakes even in places like Vermont and far up in Canada. Why? Pollution. . . . . man has nearly ruined his number one resource and survival need . . . drinking water. As a result many people have stopped drinking water unconciously without realizing it.

"Impure water, a Growing Hazard to the Health of Millions," says a headline in the *New York Times*, 5/13/73, in a seven-column feature story that continues by vividly describing what many of us already feared . . . our drinking water and cooking water at home, in recreation vehicles, at vacation areas, in public restaurants, is badly polluted and contaminated, and is getting worse. The story names areas of the country where already water is condemned.

From the baby's first cry to the old man's last breath, we all need water every day. Water is the one element you need the most and suspect the least! If this shocks you, do not be surprised. Millions of Americans are still unaware of the danger to our aging process and to illness. Multitudes suffer from arthritis, cataracts, diabetes, emphysema, gall stones, glaucoma, hardening of the arteries, kidney stones, loss of hearing, and obesity. Somehow the help of shots, pills, vitamins, balanced diets, as a rule add only brief spurts to our well being.

Distilled water is the greatest solvent on earth . . . *the only one that can be taken into the body without damage to the tissues.* By continued use, it is possible to dissolve minerals, acid crystals, and all the other water in the body without injuring tissue. The reason pure H_2O with nothing added to interfere with our biochemical processes.

After mineral deposits are dissolved in water, gentle muscular exercise can force the dissolved poisons and wastes from the tissues into the blood, by solvent action, so the blood can carry such wastes to the excretory organs. Then those organs can pour and squeeze the wastes out of the body.

Remember the great scientists now, not only admit, but assert, that old age, and even death, (unless by accident) is due to *waste poisons 'not' washed out of the body.*

What we have never realized is that these collected minerals, from the air, and in the ground, are all inorganic minerals . . . which *cannot* be assimilated by the body. The only minerals the body can utilize are *organic* minerals. All other minerals are foreign substances and must be disposed of or eliminated. Herein lies the problem we never suspected, a cause of nearly all our aging diseases. All the water that passes through the roots of plants converts the *inorganic* minerals and distills the water at the same time, but not in the human body.

The truth of drinking distilled water is not new. The U.S. Navy has been using it for decades; distilled water is used in intravenous feeding, inhalation therapy, prescriptions, and baby formulas, because it has a known formula without chemical contamination. All kidney machines operate on distilled water. And since the body is made up of 70% water, we should be a little particular about what water goes into our body. But it is just that the public has never caught on; they took water as a matter of course.

Now, here we are back on the salt discussion again. Machine-made "soft water" has salt or sodium in it. This is produced from the calcium ions (the hard water) changing by ion exchange to sodium ions. So the harder the water was before softening, the more sodium is contained in the soft water, and that isn't good. This sodium can upset our potassium-sodium electrolyte balance. When this balance is disrupted the heart cannot conduct electrical stimulus that

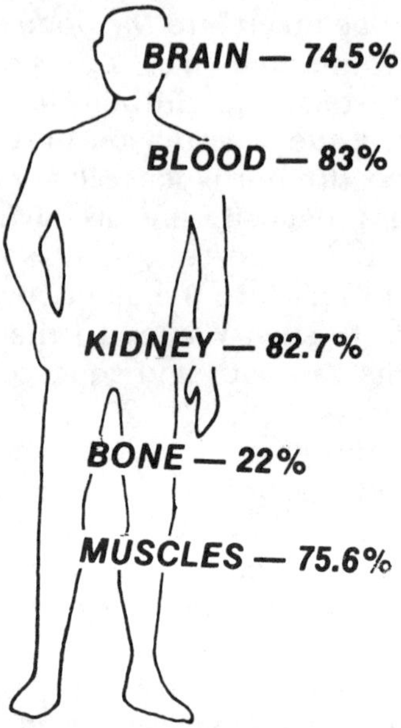

The tissues, organs, fluids and bone of the human body have a large water content.

causes the heart to beat properly; an irregular beat of the heart or heart failure results.

There has been much research done all over the world on waters rich in calcium and magnesium (hard water) and the longer life spans of those drinking it as opposed to those people living in soft water areas. In fact, the harder the water, the lower the heart disease rate. Dr. Leland Mc Cabe, Director of Epidemilogy and Biometrics of water supplies programs, divisions of the U.S. Environmental Protection Agency expounded on such facts.

Soft water, treated or untreated has calcium and magnesium in it.

Hard water has less calcium and magnesium in it.

Distilled water has nothing in it but pure H2O.

Soft water has been linked with heart disease with a report dating back to 1857 in Japan. There have been hundreds of comparisons made including the U.S. Geological Survey in 1961. Results all showed the harder the water, the lower the average heart disease rates.

After finding that almost 65 Percent of Americans drink soft water, the EPA determined that 15 percent of those heart disease deaths could have been prevented by drinking hard water. If this estimate is accepted, it means that close to 10 percent of all heart disease in the U.S. could be prevented by using hard water.

Chlorine, (not chloride) like bleach (Chlorox), is a strong oxidizing agent. It affects blood vessels seriously. It destroys vitamin E in your system. Your municipal source of water most always contains chlorine.

Water from your municipal supply can contain carcingenic compounds like poisons, herbicides, and pesticides. Many carcigenic compounds are not removed by conventional municipal treatment. When water comes from a river it usually contains minute toxic sewage usually dumped in upriver somewhere. Of the 12,000 chemicals on the market today, and nearly 500 more being added yearly, is it any wonder the EPA (environmental Protection Agency) has their hands full monitoring water for pollution-causing chemicals? Likewise it is difficult to test for all these chemicals; there are just too many.

The EPA has, among others, discovered any number of chlorinated carcinogens in our drinking water. Chlorine used to treat the water to kill germs is an insidious poison, and there have been reported epidemics of heart attack and stroke as a result of high chlorine content in some city waters.

Niagara Falls, New York area, the Love Canal, recently had a serious waste dumping problem more serious than just carcinogens that caused untold health and birth problems there. It was so bad that the government moved people out of their homes to other safe places permanently.

If you have any doubts of the chlorine problem, look at Japan. They no longer chlorinate their water; their heart disease rate is one-sixth of ours.

The affluent or left-over water from sewage disposal plants is supposed to be pure and drinkable. If the sewage plant is overtaxed, this may not be possible. This always seems to be a problem here in Florida from the constant growth of homes and businesses. Anyone could have the problem. Nutrient-rich affluent prevents the natural life of water plants and animals from getting the proper oxygen they need. Algae or other plant life robs or smothers the life-giving oxygen.

What can water contain besides H_2O (that's two parts hydrogen and one part oxygen)? Such things as calcium, magnesium, sulfur, copper, iron, chlorine, solid matter, dirt, rust, slime, algae . . . to name a few; none of which you can see, some of which you can taste.

Well water, usually suspect today, may contain anything and everything that travels and penetrates through layers of soil with the rainfall. It cannot be filtered out completely by the earth so it is deposited finally in our water below the earth.

Besides impurities in most waters, today we have various kinds of water available to us. Some we may be familiar with. Let's run them down:

Chlorinated water or city water is usually normal drinking water from the municipal supply system treated with chlorine that is added to kill bacteria. Some cities add flouride to prevent tooth decay. This is "sodium" floride. This can be soft or hard. It is not good for the body or your heart. Chlorine is a bleach and is poison that affects the blood vessels seriously, with gradual destruction. It destroys Vitamin E and one of the "E" vitamins' uses is just to counteract the effects of chlorine; so we must take "E" in larger doses.

Purified water is a "catch-all" word and is suspect. It is usually sold in jugs and large dispensers. If water is passed through charcoal of sufficient quantity, it is filtered. Gadgets sold on TV and in stores that fit on your faucet are charcoal filters. They are too small. If water passes through charcoal that is impregnated with silver ions it can kill bacteria also. The astronauts drink from this NASA system. This water can be soft or hard, depending on who purifies it and what else they do to treat the water.

Spring water is another "catch-all" word. Many years ago spring water meant water from a mountain spring. It was usually uncluttered, and since it was cold, it tasted very good. People used to take jugs to the spring and bring home the water for drinking and cooking. It is sold today in bottles and *may* come from a spring. Again, if it is cold, it usually tastes good without you knowing just what is in it.

Bottled water is another "catch all" word for water sold in stores that could be spring water, mineral water, purified water, or some sort of treated water, even local tap water.

Mineral water is from certain areas where minerals are plentiful in the water or where the effects are therapeutic in value to some people. Perrier water, recently introduced in our market, is from Perrier, France. It is expensive and used as a carbonated water of "mixer" in drinks. It is a mineral water and naturally carbonated. It, too, tastes better served cold.

Distilled water is pure 100 percent water (if distilled thoroughly): no hardness, no softness, no carcigens, almost nothing but clean pure water. If it is purchased it could be suspect in its claims as there are no regulations on the quality standards of water. The best idea and the cheapest is to distill your own water, which in turn will have you drink more of it. It can be distilled in the home conveniently for 10-15 cents per gallon.

Some say distilled water tastes flat compared to what they were drinking before . . . that could be true. But distilled water really has no taste at all; all the junk has been removed which gives the water the "distinctive flavor," if anything. You will discover that a glass of cold, distilled water tastes "*clean*". What's more, the flavors or anything you mix with the water such as coffee, tea, or fruit juice, taste better; there is nothing left in the distilled water to interfere with or change the original natural flavor of the mix.

Now you say, how about the minerals you take out of the water? Very simple . . . just go on eating foods, many of which contain minerals to satisfy this need; and man's needs are minimal but steady in the body. There is not one mineral that cannot be found easily in the food we eat.

Intravenous feeding is made from distilled water as is used in chelation therapy, inhalation therapy, and kidney dialysis.

Reverse osmosis is forcing water through a membrane and is a distillation process to remove most all impurities and solids. Charcoal filters, used first, help the process depending on what water purity you desire as a result. It is mostly an industrial process for large quantities of water. If it could be found in a package for the home, I believe I would have one in mine.

It is my intention to have a charcoal filter with silver ions and a reverse osmosis unit if it can be found, as this unit should remove about 98 percent of the impurities needed to be removed from water. Watch for this announcement in the back pages of this book, as this may be more convenient and almost as good as a slow water distillation process.

Water quality and water scarcity are destined to be our two big problems of the 1980s. Chemical pollution could be our #1 environmental issue in the 1980, says Robert H. Harris, of president Carter's Council on Environmental Quality. "Sixty Minutes" just recently dramatized the pollution effects on water quality to our rivers and streams. The issue is heating up, here's why:

- Our clues to the aging process of people is determined in part by our water quality.
- Illness and disease are caused in part by poor water quality.
- If pollution grows worse, so will our quality of life.
- The population explosion and the scarcity of water will be with us to the end of the century at least.
- Our new chemical product development and other large users of water will be affected and affect the scarcity and quality.
- Our water table is slowly nearing the critical stage and the absence of rainfall can be dangerous.
- In our complex bodies we still have not found all the answers to our biological process of life. So far we seem to take clues to problems of illness and present answers as much as is reasonibly possible. The environmental quality of water and air should be our primary concern.

But water is so good for you and your body and your health . . . you can see now it is a vital subject. In fact, the next chapter adds to the seriousness of the pure water problem.

I am told that you should drink half your weight in ounces of water daily. If you weigh 160 pounds you should drink 80 ounces of water per day. 120 pounds needs 60 ounces of pure water per day. Not many people drink this much water, so they may doubt authentic recommendation.

Water also fills your stomach, which means you eat less if there's less room for food. If you take your vitamin pills right before eating, there's less room for food.

But more importantly, our concern is that water washes away waste products by its solvent or detergent action from fat metabolism. Better get on the clean water wagon. The choice is clear . . . water.

SUMMARY THOUGHT!

A peek into the future is bleak and discouraging. Water more precious than oil? Water is more appreciated where it is scarce. Look around you for answers to problems close at home. "Waste not-want not" could turn into "do not waste" or "do not use."

Chapter Twenty-Two

MAKING PREVENTION PAY OFF

"One thing common to most sucess stories is the alarm clock."
. . . Anon.

During the past decades we have pretty much resolved our past problems such as infectious disease. We developed hygiene, antibiotics and immunization. This left a small gap in the development of certain virus' since we have not yet found all antibodies, or, our bodies have not built up its own immune system. We do have answers to about 80 percent of heart disease and stroke but this still needs our immediate attention. This then leaves old number two, cancer, sticking out like a sore thumb, and where we should really concern ourselves with. We now know that aging is not an old man's disease and it can be reversed. We know that circulation, nutrients and oxygen carried in the blood has a direct relationship to many diseases as well as heart disease. Yes we have answers, but we also have problems, for instance.

Medical research is tied pretty much to conventional medicine. We shall call it the old faction. They have built emphasis on crisis care or treatment of symptoms, the one avenue of medicine they know well. But this involves treating the end results of disease. Other than administering prescription drugs and surgery, very little has been done to *PREVENT* patients with real but seemingly minor complaints from progressing into a more recognizable degenerative disease. Isn't it time we started to recognize warning stages or risks of forthcoming medical problems, to ward off an eventual illness that brings with it financial crisis in health care expenses as well as suffering?

After all we do have alternative groups of modern

medical practitioners we call the new faction, who are now performing a real and successful medical service to many people.

Here we have two separate opposing groups of medical practitioner, both fighting to obtain a more prominent place in the world of medicine.

The dispute is hardly known to the public and kept pretty much hidden under the rug by the AMA's powerful influence. Simply and basically described I see the old generation of medicine represented by the AMA and the new generation of emerged modern professional with fresh new ideas. These the two opposing factions. I see outmolded ineffective treatment versus new very effective techniques.

I see Goliath power trying to trample down the David of practicality. I see the same Goliath a victim of self overkill, slain from the seed he sprouted as it came into full bloom. I see the result from monoply, excessive charges and greed struck down in a victory by this modern practical professional.

After thirty years and trillions of dollars later, spent on research by the older faction, they produce little in answers to cancer and heart disease. In comparison this book speaks with pride of the successes of the new breed of professional. Someone should step in and straighten out this serious mess.

We have arrived at an opportune time for a national prevention program. We have expert knowledge, all the records and experiences of the world at hand, and the modern tools to implement preventive measures today. Now.

It is just as simple to predict an illness and take measures of prevention rather that to pospone the illness by the delayed action of a drug. We have all the tools needed within our present knowledge and grasp. Prevention is proven every day and has for years, preventive physicians have made many people well. But like any successful technique history records violent dissent. The "in's versus the "out's. The subject has come up before and the powerful in's are able squelch the idea and publicity early. But this preventive medical field is growing fast and so successful that dissent may be abating. Herein lies the solution to our medical problems.

Looking at cancer, it is estimated that 80 to 90 percent of human cancer may be related to enviromental factors.

Nutrition and diet are included in those factors. Caloric restriction, the amount of dietary fat by type, vitamin and mineral deficiencies, the dietary content of protein and amino acids, all influence induction or growth of tumors in animals. High levels of fat and lack of fiber in the diet is a causation of breast and colonic cancer. Cancer of the bowel can be affected by micro-bacteria variations.

In the last several years hypoglycemia has been an important popular diagnosis. Before this many patients were treated excessively with potentially hazardous medications along with diet restrictions, many still are treated similarly. Actually about 90 precent of these patients can be treated with diet modifications and no medication. The test is primarily for early diabetes mellitus detection and other stages of hypoglycemia and liver diseases.

So diabetes mellitus is characterized by hypoglycemia, a deficiency of insulin and other symptoms or manifestations. This is entirely reversable with treatment. Many different factors can produce diabetes and increase the risk of the disease. Obesity, genetic factors and diet are important indicators.

Cancer of the colon, lung cancer and breast cancer are the leading concerns and in that order of fatality. In order to simplify our chart that follows we have chosen as an example of predictability three major degenerative diseases to simplify our point.

The chart featured takes into account our top major diseases. It purpose is to show that all three diseases are predictable to some degree and thus preventable. There have been billions of dollars spent on research into these three diseases. So we really need only to look back at results of the research to find the basic risk factors or symptoms of each disease. When we arrive at prominant factors in numbers we also have predictability factors. Then we can arrive at prevention measures to suppress the onset of these conditions.

When scoring yourself on any disease, remember; the more risk factors present, the more likely is the possibility of that disease occurring. Each combination of factors increases the risk of say, heart disease, *by four times*. So says the famous Framingham study.

If 100 ailing people had a diagnostic physical examination by a prevention oriented, and nutritionally knowledgable

(D) RISK FACTORS →

X = RISK FACTOR
V = PART RISK

		FAMILY HISTORY CONGENITAL	HIGH BLOOD PRESSURE HYPERTENSION	OBESITY OVERWEIGHT	ENVIRONMENTAL WORK HABITS	SMOKING ALCOHOL CAFFEINE	LACK OF EXERCISE SEDENTARY LIFESTYLE	NUTRITION DEFICIENCY	STRESS – OVERWORK DEPRESSION/FRUSTRATION TEMPER	HIGH SERUM CHOLESTEROL	PROCESSED FOODS (B) NITRATES/CARCIGENS FOOD ADDITIVES	WHITE FLOUR SUGAR WHITE BREAD	INTERNAL IRRITATION CONSTIPATION
CORONARY HEART DISEASE		X	X	X	X	X	X	X	X	X	X	X	
STROKE		V	X	V	X	X	X	V	X	X	X	X	
MAIN CANCERS (C)	Cancer of Colon		X	X		X	X	X	X		X	X	X
	Lungs (A)		X	V	X	X	X	X			V	V	
	Breast		V	V	X	V		X	X	V	X	X	
DIABETES		X	X	X	X	X	X	X	X	X	X	X	V

CORRELATION IN LIFESTYLE INCIDENCE TO MAJOR DISEASES

[All Predictable and Preventable]

SCORE YOURSELF. HELP PREDICT SERIOUS ILLNESS.

NOTES:

(A) There is 10 to 30 times the risk for other cancers as a non-smoker.
(B) Only 10% of cholesterol comes from what we eat. 90% is manufactured in the body from saturated fats and refined carbohydrates.
(C) The main cause of cancer (risk factors) follow virtually the same pattern; but there are more risk factors.
(D) Compiled from various medical sources and physician questionnaire from known experience.

physician, to arrive at an indicated factor for recommending preventive steps for the patient to take. The same risk factors would be prevalent in from 50 to 70 of the 100 patients.

If we used a computer and fed that computer all the information resulting from past research; we would no doubt have uncovered the important and predominant risk factors we have arrived at in this chart. As a result, if 100 sick people had life habits fed into the computer, the computer would indicate about 75 percent of the 100 people had eight to twelve bad health habits.

It appears that heart attack and stroke then could be about 75 to 85 percent reliable or precictable. The major kinds of cancer then would be from 60 to 90 percent predictable. For a disease like cancer that people do not understantd, and some even blame on the Lord, who believe it incurable by a doctor and uncontrollable by a patient, this predictability is excellent.

The conclusion is that if these diseases are predictable and we heed the risks, it is much easier to prevent them from occurring. So we are back again to that major motivational effort, changing our lifestyle. To go with that of course, is correction of our biological problems and that is accomplished in consultation with your physician's advice with diet, exercise and proper nutrition.

There are other physicians in conflict with the AMA. Like AAMP and the Holistic Medical Association there is the Orthomolecular Medical Society. They too, in order to strengthen the body's defenses use vitamins and minerals and other nutritional methods. They treat disease by manipulating the natural body chemistry and in contrast to the AMA, they give drugs only when they must.

The founder of the Society Dr. Michael Lesser has said that disease in most cases is inborn or induced, chemical imbalance, and the nutrition we talk about is just chemistry. They don't say that drugs are bad or surgery is bad, but they do say that the physician should first try to correct the problem nutritionally. So you see that these new factions with the names preventive medicine, holistic medicine or orthomolecular medicine are one and the same. The physicians practicing this successful therapy are the center of one of medicines most heated controversies with the AMA. But like your writer who offers proof within these pages, they are making thousands of converts every day. And as Dr. Lesser mentions he needs to keep finding new patients as the old ones keep getting well.

The field of medical prevention is long overdue to be placed in the forefront of medicine even in its adolescencence stage. Thanks to Dr. Roger Williams, director of the Clayton Foundation Biological Institute at the University of Texas in Austin. Dr. Williams has worked out a list of recommendations that he calls "vitamin and mineral formulation for nutritional insurance." Most all the physicians in preventive medicine use his estimates in preference to the U.S. RDA we see on the labels of so many processed foods. Williams contributions are world famous.

Treating disease with diet is NOT something new; rather it is one of the oldest in medicine. Ancient people were all nutritionists. Hippicroates, the father of medicine 2500 years ago said "let thy food by thy medicine and thy medicine thy food". Maimonides, in the 13th century said "Let nothing that can be treated by diet be treated by any other means."

Dr. Bernard Rimland, has been most critical of the AMA and their use of drugs and tranquilizers and says that modern medicine is bankrupt and is making a nighmare for people as many advances have backfired. They have caused blindness stroke, and physician caused diseases more serious than the original disease. He said as a result that prescription drugs now equal breast cancer as a leading cause of death in this country.

For those readers interested in further enlightening comments and arguments I recommend reading "ORTHOHEALING", by Belinda Dumont in OMNI Magazine Feb. 1980.

The body and mind are one; its all Y-O-U in person. If you are not doing right for one, you are not helping the whole person. Any malfunction affects the person directly or indirectly and contineous malfunction is disease.

There is a natural knowledge inside all of us as to what we know is best for us, but we have forgotten.

Now we have to strengthen this knowledge with a defense against media advertising telling us how good that certain food is for us. We are bombarded by self-serving opinion, by government, and by the fast food industry. Isn't it time to reason with ourselves, examine our lifestyles, ponder the differences from the history of our healthy past and make changes we need?

People are still getting sick. There's no marked decrease in disease today. All the research we have done over the past thirty years, all the contributions we have made to the American Cancer Society and the American Heart Association, and all the billions of dollars the government has poured into these causes, has not helped markedly to cure anything. There seems to be small discoveries or clues that may help but realistic accomplishments are not forthcoming. It has cost us trillions of dollars already but to no avail. Our survival is at stake now not only health-wise but financially.

Conventional medicine is deeply involved as they are beneficiaries of power and prestige, in employment and research resources not only of the cancer and heart charities, but also of government directly supported National Institute of Health, National Cancer Institute, The National Heart, Lung and Blood Institute, The National Institute on Aging to name only a few. Is it any wonder then that they continue on the same theories of treatment, when they benefit directly from such policies. They are in one word, CONTROL over our medical destiny.

This chart shows how a combination of three major risk factors can increase the likelihood of heart attack. For purposes of illustration, this chart uses an abnormal blood pressure level of 180 systolic, and a cholesterol level of 310 in a 45-year old man.

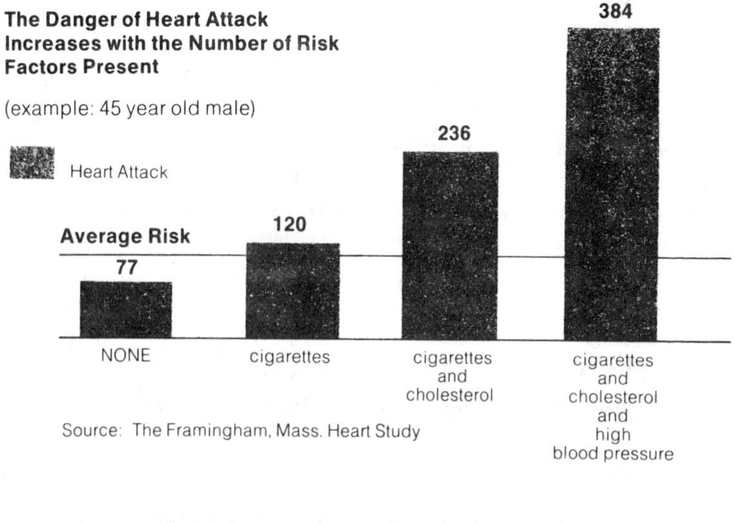

We have a positive approach in prevention, this is not some new idea, its older than most of us. The statistics have been established for predictability and prevention. At this crucial stage in the game its the cheapest insurance we could buy for ourselves and our children.

Its time to fill this obvious void in our health delivery system by early diagnosis and treatment of subtle but demonstrational metabolic abnormalities that are known to precede and manifest diseases. In this way we lessen the tragic toll of most degenerative diseases.

SUMMARY THOUGHT!

The salvation of sick people saved from the power of conventional medicine, lie in the ailing heart of our social system. The answer is prevention of disease.

Chapter Twenty-Three

NATIONAL HEALTH REFORMATION IS FOR YOU.

"You believe that easily which you hope for earnestly."
. . . Terence

This *is* something new! With God's help we will hear a great deal more about prevention of our health problems, so that we may nip our minor ills in the bud before they become serious. And so that the new administration in Washington can be influenced to promote a national prevention program at NO COST to the government or taxpayers.

In essence, it is a program to:

- Educate citizens to the importance of new health habits, exercise and nutrition.
- Foster economic competition in hospitals such as HMO prepaid health plans; and P.M. diagnostic clinics with built in incentives to keep the citizens well.
- To drastically cut the cost of health care by prevention, early diagnosis and thus save billions of dollars yearly.
- Relax the rules laid down by Congress and enforced by the FDA of many needed medical breakthrough's and drugs being suppressed by the FDA for many years.
- Eliminate bureaucratic control or pay the costs of medical research as it restricts initiative and lowers the quality of medical services.

- To allow the administration of chelation therapy not only as a corrective clinical therapy, but also to prevent heart disease and many other maladies.
- Help originate a network of private preventive diagnostic clinics. To spot and help eradicate major diseases by computer predictability and prevention information of facts already well known, for any person seeking this information.

Sponsor a media campaign of DISEASE IS PREDICTABLE AND PREVENTABLE.

In my opinion and that of many knowledgable experts, such a program would cost the government little or nothing. It will literally save billions of dollars yearly in social security disability payments as well as Medicare and Medicaid payments, just as starters.

History has shown that we cannot count on that segment of the medical profession that supports AMA policies. First of all, the majority of such physicians have had little or no education in diet and nutrition. Secondly, there is no money in prevention or they would have been in it long ago. Third, they will no doubt oppose these ideas as theyhave in the past.

Such a physician is like the auto mechanic working on your car. He's interested in replacing parts as they cause problems, and you can get an occasional tune-up. He does nothing on preventive maintenance because there's no money in it for him.

In my own case I now know that my heart attack could have been prevented. Had I known about symptoms and risks in advance, I would have had a chance to avoid the problem. I had already received the "hints" from my body, the indigestion like pain while pushing the lawn mower. Had I been knowledgable that the pain was an alarming symptom, I could have taken steps to prevent the heart attach from happening. How many victims could have been saved, that had fewer symptoms that could have been prevented?

I am assured that an efficiently run preventive diagnostic clinic, aided by the latest computerized and diagnostic equipment to evaluate and plot each patients medical future, would be self-supporting. An attending physician, several medical technicians and two clerks could handle a minimum of 32 patients per day.

Since it would be self supporting financially, the beneficiary would be the patient and the elimination of cost to government of expensive *"crisis care."*

But let's digress a little at this point. Let's dream up a little fiction to bring out my point of view from my experience.

I (should have) made an appointment with the P.M. diagnostic Health Clinic located nearby. The government advertisement said that diesase and most illness is predictable and preventable and that it is less costly to be healthy. It made a great deal of sense. My modern medical examination would be most thorough and they would be able to tell me their recommendations on ways to be healthy after diagnosis is completed. They can predict disease years in advance. They can spell out in writing for future reference a complete detailed report for the patient to follow.

They set the cost of this complete fee at $200. For those qualified under Medicare this is paid on the usual 80/20 percent arrangement. Private insurance carriers would surely conform. This leaves the less fortunate citizen who would have to pay a part and the government subsidize the balance from benefits effected from the savings.

I am sure I would have a great deal to gain from this public program developed by private funds and supported by the government. I will have a high degree of health, I am free to seek the suggested treatment from experienced physicians in that phase of medical expertise, I have avoided a heart attack, any my insurance costs would be lowered by my improved health experience.

If I failed to heed the recommendations of the clinic I would be warned at the preappointed next visit. Upon further disregard for recommendations I would lose all rights to government subsidy in the future.

As a preventive therapy, anyone whose tests indicate a build-up of obstructive plaque in the arteries can be recommended for preventive chelation therapy treatments. If that person reverts back to his former lifestyle again upon a check-up he is warned in a similar way.

In the clinic on a computerized form, I reveal all my living and eating habits, my past medical history and that of my family. My past and current medical problems are recorded, I have a hair analysis and nutritional analysis. I would be given a series of non-invasive tests to determine my present and future health status. The lab technicians and the computer would evaluate results and feed them into the central computer. The results would be sent back to the clinic physician so that he would know in advance which areas of concern would need further evaluation and attention for that patient. Then after examination, the physicians findings would be fed back into the central computer.

The results of all the tests, the physicians findings and personal evaluations made by the patient are all evaluated by the computer. This will be compared to the logic and statistics stored in the computer memory resulting from information from the best representation of medical experience in the world.

A word processor will produce the results and recommendations in hard copy for the benefit of me the patient, for the physician who is to perform the recommended therapy and for future records. The patient takes home the sheath of findings so he can study them in detail and implement them as needed.

I am sure that if I had such a thorough extensive evaluation and, diagnosis into my past bad habits explained to me in such a respected and elaborate manner, I would have been impressed. That such far flung knowledge stored and used for my personal benefit, was important enough for me to follow to the letter.

If I was forwarned and heeded the PM Clinic's advice, I not only would *NOT* have had a heart attack but the government and I would have saved $6826. on hospitalization and post treatment care. For a fee of $200. this saving would be directly evaluated at about $6600. Indirectly the dollar benefit in absenteeism, suffering, and family strain and hundreds of other events blamed on my health problem probably equals that amount again or more.

Its time to have everyone realize why we are getting sick, why disease, and why people are dying off so fast. Look at our physical bodies; they haven't changed in more than two hundred years. We eat the same way, digest the same way,only we don't eat the same foods or exercise as much. Our bodies were never meant to undergo stress and the conflicts of the fast-paced world. We just don't have the metabolic machinery inside us to keep up efficiently to the intake of Modern age foods that we eat and their resulting problems. Our environment has changed. These fact's must be known to everyone.

HERE ARE HIGHLIGHTS FOR NATIONAL HEALTH REFORMATION DIAGNOSTIC PROGRAM.

A central computer will be fed medical data of informational statistics from a broad source of renowned medical, government and educational sources. This would leave little room for error when comparisons are made by each branch clinic terminal.

All the preventive measures you have read about previously will be included as well as thousands of data on eating habits, exercise and normal lifestyles. Age, height, weight, body structure and physical condition will also be included.All data compared to each individual patients report as it is fed in to the computer for comparisons.

By using a comprehensive group of facts from scientific and medical brains, programmed into the computer and later compared with tests and analysis at the clinic with programmed norms, we have some valuable information for the patient. Hence your body chemistry factory is placed on a successful, proven guided path for future health.

The physician in charge of the clinic examines the computer results of pre-tests and questionaires so far, PRIOR to his examination of the patient. He has computer clues as to what to look for in a close medical examination. After the examination the physicians results are fed back into the computer, where they are again assimilated and recognized and finally determined for each patient. The final results are then printed out for each patients personal records.

Its time to recognize that in this age of automation it is to our advantage to make the most of modern electronics. This progress in supplying medical help to those who need it at the lowest possible price in an automated way, from the best brains in the world is indeed a bargain at any price.

BENEFITS OF A NATIONAL HEALTH REFORMATION PROGRAM

VALUABLE TIME SAVED. More patients can be examined and served per day to keep costs low. Such a program could be almost completely automated to the capacity of the personnel, testing equipment and examination. The physicians job is mainly examination, analysis and overall supervision of the clinic. No medical treatment is performed.

MONEY IS SAVED. Computer analysis has already been proved in savings of time, money and the storing of complicated knowledge. The lengthy lag time between test, analysis and later results are saved. Unneeded recall and return the second time for receiving results is eliminated for personnel and patient saving.

ACCURACY OF INFORMATION. I would rather have 100 professional opinions and diagnosis than just one or two. The world-wide facts in consensus must be superior to any confusion of opinions and alternatives normally used.

PRINT—OUTS FOR PATIENTS. there is little chance of error or misunderstanding when all the final information for the patient is issued in printed form.

CLINIC ECONOMIC STRUCTURE. This could be financed in part by government loans, with private capital investment, and to private qualified medical professionals. The entire investment could be paid back over a nominal period from starting funds of government and private capital. Leases would be from the owner of the central computer to leasing terminals at each clinic. Reasonable profits can be effected by present fees commensurate with each clinic's responsibilities and efficiency; so much so that low flat fees would be inviting to any person.

POSSIBLE CITIZEN SAVINGS COMPARISONS

CHART NUMBER ONE

ALTERNATIVE A. . . . *My personal record of medical expense, no drugs, from my heart attack, under Medicare.*

I DESCRIPTION	I PAID	MEDICARE EXPENSE	TOTAL
Hospital, doctor, diagnostic, cath test in hospital.	592.	3,017.	3,609.
Post treatment, doctor, chelation therapy (b)	2,967.	250. (b)	3,217.
TOTAL FOR HEART ATTACK CORRECTION	3,559.	3,267.	6,826.
ALTERNATIVE B. . . . *Bypass surgery substitution for chelation therapy (est.)*			
Initial heart attack same as above	592.	3,017.	3,609.
Post treatment and bypass surgery. (estimates)	3,750.	14,920.	18,650.
TOTAL FOR HEART ATTACK CORRECTION	5,342.	17,937.	22,259.

TOTAL chelation therapy versus bypass surgery, savings by chelation $16,433

NOTE: "b" chelation therapy is not a recognized procedure as yet, treatment payments are refused. Initial examination is paid by Medicare.

Estimates have been arrived at by inquiry and quotation by surgeon quotation given me by actual patients, all averaged.

A further extension on this estimate concerns the American Heart Association estimate of 80,000 bypass operations performed yearly.

Yearly savings

. . . . 80,000 operations yearly X $16,433.
= Savings by Chelation Therapy = $13,146,4000.

CHART NUMBER TWO

ESTIMATED PREVENTION SAVINGS FROM CORONARY VASCULAR DISEASE

BASED **ONLY ON BYPASS SURGERIES PERFORMED.**	**VARIOUS PREVENTION SAVINGS ESTIMATES**		
American Heart Assoc. estimate 80,000 yearly. NOT INCLUDING non-operative cases.	YEARLY SAVINGS		
From chart #1 cost of surgery & treatment . . . 22,259.00 each.	20% save =	40% savings	60% savings
$22,259. each X 80,000 = 17,807,200.	3,554,440.	7,122,880.	10,684,320.

SUMMARY: National Health Reformation can cut from 3.5 million to 10.7 million from just bypass procedures alone. The three estimates given as an start to the NHR program with increases in future years increasing more than estimates. To eventual near elimination of the procedure.

Chelation therapy used in conjunction with NHR prevention measures could virtually wipe out this problem in ten years.

CHART NUMBER THREE

ESTIMATED PREVENTION MEASURE SAVINGS
FROM CORONARY VASCULAR DISEASE

BASED ON AMERICAN HEART ASSOCIATION	**VARIOUS PREVENTION SAVINGS ESTIMATES**		
ESTIMATE OF $40.8 BILLION	20% save =	40% save =	60% save =
DOLLARS SPENT IN 1980 ON C.V.D (CardioVascular Disease.)			
TOTAL 40.8 billion dollars	8.16	16.24	24.48
Of this total **consumers spent** . . : 50.3 percent	4.105	8.21	12.36
Source: Social Security Administration Chart #145 on Expendatures			
GOVERNMENT SPENT 40.6 percent	3.13	6.62	9.94

SUMMARY: On this basis of dollars spent on coronary vascular disease. National Health Reformation could conservatively cut from 8.16 billion to 24.48 billion on coronary vascular disease in the beginning years.

CHART NUMBER FOUR

PROJECTED HEALTH SAVINGS FROM NATIONAL HEALTH REFORMATION FROM HEALTH & HUMAN SERVICES 1982 BUDGET

The HHS budget*

ENTITLEMENTS	1980	1981	1982	Δ %
Social Security	$117.1	$138.3	$159.6	15.4%
Medicare ✓	35.0	39.9	**46.0**	17.0%
Medicaid ✓	13.9	16.5	**18.1**	9.7%
Aid to Families with Dependent Children	7.3	7.8	7.7	− 1.3%
Supplemental Security Income	6.4	7.3	8.0	9.6%
Benefits for Coal Miners	1.0	1.1	1.1	—
Title XX Social Services	2.8	3.1	3.1	—
Other	.1	.1	.1	—
Subtotal	$183.6	$214.1	$244.3	14.1%
Percentage of Total	93.7%	94.2%	94.6%	
DISCRETIONARY FUNDS				
Health Programs ✓	$ 7.7	$ 7.9	$ **8.2**	3.8%
Low-Income Energy Assistance	1.6	1.8	1.8	—
Human Development Services (principally Head Start and Aging programs)	2.2	2.2	2.7	22.7%
Refugee and Entrant Assistance	.5	.9	.8	−11.1%
Other	.3	.4	.4	—
Subtotal	$ 12.3	$ 13.2	$ 13.9	5.3%
Percentage of Total	6.3%	5.8%	5.4%	
Total, HHS Outlays	$195.9	$227.3	$258.2	13.6%

*Outlays in billions

Source: Dept. of Health and Human Services

CITIZENS AND GOVERNMENT ESTIMATED SAVINGS FROM NATIONAL HEALTH REFORMATION

ESTIMATES FROM CHART. HEALTH & HUMAN SERVICES 1982 budget.

The above HHS Budget chart illustrates various entitlements in the projected budget for 1982 as determined by Secretary Richard Schweiker's department. Only three major illness / disease related costs are in the areas of consideration here. They are Medicare, Medicaid, and Health programs, for consideration in this chart.

Medicare at ....46.8 billion dollars.
Medicaid at ....18.1 billion dollars.
Health Programs at ..... 8.2 billion dollars.

TOTAL COST OF THESE THREE PROGRAMS .... 72.9 billion dollars.

20.5% of total Social Security Budget.

SUPPOSTION: If we prevent illness, hospital costs and cut the health programs need because of National Health Reformation; and use the same percentage of savings estimates contained on previous charts, we arrive at results as follows:

	ESTIMATED STARTING YEARS OF PREVENTION SAVINGS. YEARLY SAVINGS		
	20% save =	40% save =	60% save =
MEDICARE / MEDICAID CITIZENS GOVERNMENT COST .....72.9 billion .... Charge is 80% of total bill	14.58	29.26	43.74
CITIZENS COSTS ADD TO ABOVE .... (20% paid by citizens)	2.91	5.83	8.74
TOTAL GOVERNMENT AND CITIZENS COST.	17.49	24.99	52.48

NOTE: This does ***not include ALL CITIZENS***, only those covered by Medicare

ASSUMPTION: take 40% added to the above costs by government and we arrive at or close to our annual medical care costs.	$174.96 billion dollars		
Carrying the estimates still farther we have	7.0	10.0	31.4
Estimated savings then from same estimates TOTAL ALL CITIZENS	24.49	60.00	84.52

ALL FIGURES BILLIONS OF DOLLARS

For a National Prevention program involving so many possibilities and so many dollar amounts, we still arrive at some respectable accurate savings estimates, many of which appear to be very legitimate calculated estimates. Considering the small cost to government sponsorship, overcome by the savings themselves, we respectively believe the government can ill afford NOT to call a national conference to explore the possibilities of National Health Reformation.

Let's look at some interesting facts worth considering in light of this proposal for National Health Reformation and the prevention of disease:

FACT *The surgeon General has staggering figures on health care costs. Last year, 1980 under President Carter he called for a look at prevention in medicine. The report was "Health Promotion and Disease Prevention."*

FACT *The drug industry is complaining about their rising costs while waiting approval of new product review by the FDA. It seem each individual delay means a widening gap from an average of two years to six to ten years. Premarketing costs have skyrocketed from 6 million to $70 million for new drug introduction. The article states it takes a huge bite from the 17 year life of a drug patent, and they need relief. Here is one* *government problem creating another problem that costs people more money for drugs as a result of FDA delay.*

FACT *A social Security study states that disability claims may be in error. The article states that 19.3 percent of the $17 billion disability benefits may be in error because of questionable disabilities in April 1979. This spurred another study in a effort to perfect a way to estimate waste in the program.*

Many heart disease victims already disabled can be helped by chelation therapy. Also, victims contemplating disability action as the only means they know to help them financially, can be helped by chelation and possibly prevented from becoming wards of the government. The useless life of disability is not worth the hopeless attitude, inactivity, and almost useless existance; that can be eliminated somewhat by chelation therapy. The charts indicate the savings, this comment indicates the additional savings accomplished by putting back into the workforce many disabled heart victims.

FACT *The American Cancer Society has announced that beginning in March 1981, plans for a major study of close to one million people will be undertaken to determine how their lifestyle affects the risks of getting the disease.*

The Society using volunteer workers starting in Tampa, plan to interview and record selected Americans to see what they eat, drink, smoke, how they live, work and play. The study will be monitored and recorded for six years.

In Making the announcement Dr. Edward F. Scanlon stated that it now seems clear that many people live their way into cancer. The president of the American Cancer Society, remarking on the six year study said, that by the end of the study they may have a solid basis that many of us live our way into cancer, just at people can live their way into heart disease, said the doctor.

Dr. Scanlon used the same examples of cigarette smoking to show that 100,00 cancer deaths are caused by cigarette smoking each year. But included in the study would be new questions of caffiene in coffee, and cola drinks, low tar and low nicotine in cigarettes, new consumer products and drugs, what elements of food seem to be hazardous and how birth control pills affect the risks of cancer.

It is my belief that Dr. Scanlon, the American Cancer Society and organized medicine, his own profession, have not yet recognized the wealth of statistics already established by them, and by government and preventive medicine specialists, (whom they have not recognized), or, scientists and nutritionists over the last twenty-five years into virtually the same questions.

Granted the results of the study would be revealing it seems to me to be an effort in futility (too much too late) which brings us belately up to 1987. By 1987 our medical costs will become a very critical issue leading us to fiscal bankruptcy.

If we start today with the present information already available we can accomplish virtually the same results and lead us right into a prevention program. Why wait six years? Why spend all that money and wait any longer to teach people to break these bad habits and life styles we already know about. The American Cancer Society could contribute these same earmarked funds to a cooperative effort for National Health Reformation and accomplish results several years sooner, including to boot, the saving of lives, the prevention of cancer and other diseases and its staggering costs.

FACT *Funds for government to finance medical school education are no longer needed. There are too many doctors coming out of medical school and more attention should be given to teaching nutrition in the schools.*

FACT *A Florida Senator Jack Gordon of Miami states that the biggest job of selling the government of the concept of prevention is that it is "a good buy." That the emotion of taking care of the present needs are pressing and out of necessity they may have to wait for available dollars. We hope not.*

With National Health Reformation this writer stated at

the start without any cost to government. But we will soon hear similar opposing stories and more very often, from selfish individuals and organized associations. This is a challenge to every representative in Washington. It concerns the sick, needy and those indisposed. It concerns our survival. But I can almost hear the rising indignation now as they mount their voices in selfish opposition.

The governments main job in the suggested plan, will be to foster education, the predictability and prevention of disease, and the need to go to a prevention diagnostic clinic, so important to everyone.

I can also suggest that a system is needed to reward those who keep well and penalize those who continue to dissipate and care less about their health. These no doubt, these could be the same voices rising in opposition.

Private venture capital is readily available for such an undertaking. Government can provide funding of additional loans for development of the clinic program and for publicity for implimentation. In return the government will receive much wellness from a very small investment in sponsorship, thereby reaping part of the reward in lowered health care costs and the national budget. And on the plus side of this idea. There are many congressman now in office who are already interested is such a program. Perhaps a meeting of the minds in the suggested government sponsored National Conference of **ALL medical societies and scientists**; The educational fraternities and well known scientists from Europe and Asia.

The February 23 issue of Business Week has a challenging article titled, THE STAGGERING COST OF PROLONGING LIFE, by Dr. Thomas C. Chalmers, Dean, and Dr. Alfred R. Stern, Chairman, of Mount Sinai Medical Center. It is the story of the health care system estimates to keep people functioning effectively to the end of their lives. The doctors warn our society will face a civilian form of triage because of projected ultra high and dangerous medical costs.

This is a massive problem and will worsen as the end of the centruy approaches said the authors. They state that Americans will spend more money in the next twenty years on medical care than the entire federal budget for 1980 and the doctors back their statement with support from The Health Care Financing Administration.

It is expected that health care costs will double every five years. If that doesnt startle you the facts proffered will; that by the year 2000 medical care is placed at 2.3 TRILLION DOLLARS. and by 2005 year such costs rise to 4.1 Trillion dollars. In view of these facts I don't really believe I used the term bankrupt too loosely.

The doctors advised that stop-gap measures will not do, that emphasis must be placed on prevention as the important first step. These same doctors suggest expansion and duplication of the prevention actions and therapy now going on in medicine, in nutrition and exercise. And of course like many doctors the elimination of alcohol, tobacco and carcigens from our diets.

In addition the doctors suggest we concentrate research on the processes of aging as regarding the brain. The idea is to pospone deterioration of the brain, and joints so people can keep working longer.

Their overall thought is that this will in turn diminish the financial burden on the young working class as a group in order to keep older groups working and producing longer, thereby reducing the cost of the Social Security system.

And if we don't do something the doctors say the costs of caring for the sick and disabled will be enormous. The doctors say that the scenario's they talk about may seem far-fetched but they are already happening here and abroad. It concerns the decision's being made as to who is to die and who is to live. They predict that the Congress will be talking about putting a cap on medical costs of around a trillion dollars. They also talk about decisions on the artificial heart costing $200,000. Decisions of prolonging life for six month or a year for incurable cancer. Decisions of senility costing $80,000. annually at age 104.

My opening statement on the program was "at no cost to government" or taxpayers. The benefits in dollars saved by National Health Reformation far outnumer the small investment by government in promotion, sponsorship. The raising of private capital the use of "Seed money" (loans) in attaining results that are virtually guaranteed.

And dear Reader we are talking about your government and your money that is needed to be saved by National

Health Reformation. In the rear pages is suggestions for writing your representatives in Washington. Remember the power of the numbers become effective and convincing. Isn't it little for you to do to cut your health care costs and live longer?

SUMMARY THOUGHT!

A serious thinking individual no matter his status or position in life, could hardly object to a prevention plan of any nature that directly or indirectly beneficially affects every person in this country. But the selfish interests will rise up in opposition and more importantly be overcome with rightous acclaimation and support.

Chapter Twenty-Four
THE WINNER IS YOU

"Worry is interest paid on trouble, before it falls due."
. . . William R. Inge

History and insurance actuaries, tell us about 60 percent of you readers live to be 60 years of age, but 65 percent will have heart disease, diabetes, cancer, or hypertension as your debilitating companion for the rest of your life. I am hopeful I am instrumental in reversing these facts.

In this decade of the 1980's it appears we are going to learn a great deal about scarcities. The basic subject matter changing from money and finance, wealth and poverty, to scarcity.

One basic resource we have is the limited supply of "time", human time. Each one of us has the problem, just one youth, one life to live, and time marches on too fast. We are also scarce in "human knowledge". We learn but it takes time, we only know so much and can learn new ways of doing things only so fast. Accordingly most of us face this handicap every day and it stays right with us. In other words, "we get too old fast, too late smart."

Looking at chelation therapy and national approval, it has boiled down to too many dollars needed and too much time to bring this approval to the American people. But with a great deal of faith and hope, right should win out, and the controversies should be resolved in time . . . that scarce resource.

In a preceding chapter we wrote about Dr. Ray Evers, whom I noted as "the martyr to the cause of chelation." Here again I can report that 'right wins out again." Dr. Evers problems was a subject of a Federal Trade Commision law suit against the AMA for restraint of trade. This occured during Dr. Evers harrassment and when he was forced to move into his last U.S. Clinic in Montgomery Alabama.

The following ruling is most enlightening. It seems the AMA was interested in developing innovative forms of therapy. A decision by Judge Earnest Barns, Docket #9064, dated 11/13/78, resulted from a Federal Trade Commision legal suit against the AMA and some State and County Affiliates. This is a 312-page legal summary, resulting from nine months of testimony. The Federal Court determined that "The AMA produced a formidable impediment to competition in the delivery of health care services by physicians in this country. That barrier has served to deprive consumers of free flow of information about availability of health care services, to deter the offering of innovative forms of health care, and to stifle the rise of almost every type of fee-for-service physicians in private practice. The costs to the public in terms of less expensive or even perhaps more improved forms of medical services are great."

Copies of this decision can be obtained free by writing the Bureau of Competition, Federal Trade Commision, Washington, D.C. 20580.

I remember in the lower grades of elementary school (now; that really goes way back!) "Day by day in every way I keep getting better and better." Its the same way with our problems mentioned previously. We are winning battles little by little, but we need practice, practice, practice. We need your help also.

As you read the chapter on stress, the body/mind connection, the treatment of major diseases today is increasingly seen either as psychosomatic illness or organic illness. Psychomatically, illness is said to spring from the emotions and is often dismissed as, "Oh its only in his mind."

If this is *only* in the mind we are in bad shape. Because it would be almost impossible to cure it by medicine or surgery. Accordingly, we have to call on the strength of the spirit. If as it is reported that 85 percent of our illnesses are emotionally induced, then learning how to rise up in sprit is most important.

I have been told by a true physician that medical and surgical help could be many times more consistant and possibly longer lasting if they could get people to understand there is something about them that is more physical and something more involved in their recovery than what doctors or therapy can do for them. That there is a healing process, a new dimension inside that sick person that begins to function, in the spirit, to help bring about a cure.

So we see that science has come to believe that disease is something we do to ourselves as we upset our chemical factory; accordingly we need "behavior medicine" as we treat the disease in body, mind and spirit. All equal factors in the problem that are to become equal partners in health maintanence. This is true holistic or preventive medicine. So if your doctor prescribes a tranquilizer, diet pills or other drugs, maybe its time to look elsewhere for medical help.

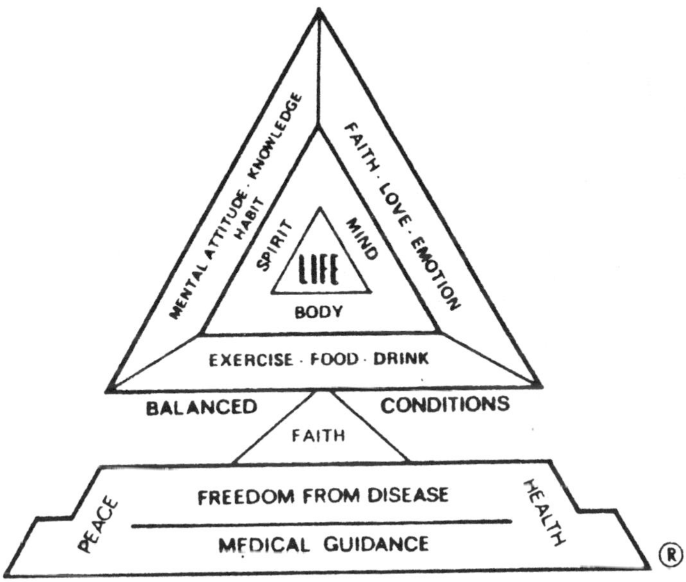

TOTAL WELLNESS, THE BODY, MIND AND SPIRIT.

Wellness is that part of life where you wake up each morning full of excitement for that day's activities, where you are cheerful and lively and full of enthusiasm for yourself and your fellow man.

Chemistry combines with the power of the mind in a wonderful partnership in a healthy body that moves the spirit to action. More than any creation, the human cells bear witness to Almighty God as Creator.

Looking at the logo on preventive medicine; an explaination will emphasize the spirit of life.

Life itself is made up of three equal parts, the body, mind and spirit, all contributing equally by their individual functions. On the body side there is the need for increased activity in exercise, and food and drink to supply nutrients to feed the body. On the mind side, you have faith and love for life and your fellow man, and, to produce emotions that instill faith and love in others. On the spirit side you have habit, mental attitude and knowledge. Habit to practice the proper mental attitude, and knowledge to gain confidence that habit and mental attitude are effective.

A consiously-controlled sense of awareness is within our so-called subconsious mind; a mental awareness to enable us to control and maintain corrected habits, enable us to activate our mind and spirit to help the body heal itself.

Expanding our mental capacities is learning to utilize the already-existing abilities within our own mind. Of particular interest is that our mind has the ability to shift awareness at will, to that area of mind function, the so called "extra sense" area, which every mind has within its capacity. Mental awareness allows the control of these inner levels of the mind, to solve the problems leading to total health.

If we are not satisfied with ourselves as we are, if we want a healthy body, we must start at the core within ourselves. Life in this core is where we can speed up or slow down the rate of action of the whole body. All this is built on faith and balanced conditions. Faith is the impelling force. "If thou cans't believe, all things are possible unto you." A strong desire backed by a firmly-held purpose, built in a powerful pyramid, is everything needed for fruition.

All this stands on a foundation that is accomplished in cooperation with your physician for medical guidance, so that you can accomplish on your own, peace of mind and a healthy body free of disease.

If we have a serious illness already, we need to change our attitudes that caused the illness in the first place, and each one of us needs to be part of this change if we are to survive. "Hope deferred makes a heart sick," says Scripture Proverb 13:12.

We need to ask ourselves some questions also. For instance, do we wish to pursue the same routine of health care that is costing us so dearly? Do we believe in ourselves, that we can change our attitude and habits that injure our health? Are we willing to still be treated for individual symptoms that may be part of the problem, and only arrest those symptoms without finding cause and correcting the cause? Should we need to depend on doctors, governments, hospitals and insurance companies to control our own destiny? Should we need to return again and again for more drugs and still more drugs?

It seems to me that it is more important that we all develop and promote our own vigorous health partnership with a knowledgable physician, to discover any of our own negative influences on our health. Education and professional influence is here today, what we need is the motivation and will to be healthy.

I see TIME Magazine reports that the AMA has adopted some sweeping changes in its ehtics code. This august body which has opposed and fought any change during its long history, has been receiving "clues" recently, and has decided to revise the code that they operate under.

This is only the first change in 23 years, and only the fifth in 133 years of its existence. There's no doubt that they have been reading and watching in detail about the state of the people's health.

They have strengthened the confidentiality of the physican/patient relationship and call for self-policing in weeding out incompetent and unethical members. The AMA has intimated to unethical practices and incompetent membership, in a statement by Dr. James Todd.

They acknowledge for the first time the substantial role of the "third party" in setting health policies. That is the government, Blue Cross and Blue Shield and other insurance underwriters. They still call it interference and they admit they now have to cope with another group, telling them what they can do on payment of claims.

They have dropped their ban on advertising, but this was ordered by the Federal Trade Commission. They have dropped the age-old rule directing doctors not to solicit the patients business. They have lifted their ban on "association" professionally with members who practice different methods of treatment such as chiropractors.

Spokesman for the AMA readily admit they were politically aware of change and that there is danger that they would be "out of step" with the times without these changes. To be more realistic their membership has dropped considerblly over the last 25 years to now 38 percent of licensed physicians.

Consumerism, increased scrutiny by the government, and the new health care groups that have been springing up in competition have shaken the AMA's dominance says Time magazine. The mammoth cost of litigation against these same groups is costing the AMA three-quarters of a million dollars a year in legal fees. This appears to continue as the State of New York has charged in a suit that the AMA interferes with freedom of medical practice. Were the AMA to lose pending law suits the Association could go bankrupt, states TIME MAGAZINE.

This appears to be the prime time for readers and consumers to rise up and join the fight. To get the AMA off the backs of the people's right to select chelation therapy (or any other therapy), an inexpensive prevention treatment for circulatory problems and heart disease.

With well over two million treatments behind them and still going strong chelation therapy physicians will get a break-through soon. The adamant stand of the FDA and their double-blind studies will change, they surely know there is no placebo for heart disease. They cannot stand very long on such a weak theory. Something will "give" soon.

In previous chapters we discussed the AMA restricting entry into medical school. Now in the early eighties ther are economic signs of turbulence among the medical practicioners. Here are the reason:

(1) New medical schools have opened and with the old schools are turning out about 16,000 doctors a year. It is predicted the doctor glut will take over soon.

(2) The boom, some $220 billion a year in medical bills, it cost us is about to turn into a bust, and it appears the business volume of many doctors will soon be threatened.

(3) The FTC is finally taking an investigative interest in Health Maintanence Organizations (HMO) and health in-

surance, and so called third party carriers. Since medical costs have zoomed unabated, private and public insurance systems had no reason to hold back the inflationary increases, thus approval and payment was a rubber stamp proposition. Now the FTC has stepped in and many offenders have agreed to back down when threatened with government legal action.

Finally there are signs and thinking that there must be a way to do it more cheaply. So there is new interest in the *cost* of health care.

(4) People are sick and tired of being sick and tired. They are getting the health food message, the bad white stuff message, the processed food message and the vitamin supplement message.

(5) It appears that many surgical procedures will be eliminated or reduced becase of economical thinking that is invading health care and poor cost/benefit ratios. Bypass operations will surely be one of them. A $2 billion bill for this operation alone is just too high when you also consider that doctors in Europe perform just seven operations for each 100 done here in this Country.

(6) There's no reason that medical findings should be secrets, shared only by those with a formal medical education. Medicine must change because life itself changes. Medicine must be challenged by the high costs; patients are no longer willing to say "doctor knows best."

In my travels I have talked to hundreds of people in the over-50 group. Most of these folks unconsiously or consiously literally are slowing down in life. They are taking dangerously, too many drugs, seeing and believing too many doctors, watching too much television (and commercials) for their own self-inflicted problems.

Many believe they are in a slow health decline, that the pills they take in increasing numbers and variety are sustaining their health, even in their declining years, and that their present lifestyle is in line with their general health. Present scientific research disputes all this "thinking."

For your own welfare I suggest it is time to analyze yourself; your food and lifestyle habits. In general, your chronic illnesses, your depressions, your sedentary life, your psychological responses, or, are you too busy "just living" to make a better life for yourself?

You should consider changing your current thinking, because if you think you are on a decline, you will BE on a decline. If you think you are beaten, you are. If you dare not to change, you don't. And if you think you can't, you won't.

Its no sin to decline in health, to go broke, to be led down the wrong road of life, because sometimes you have to *SQUAT DOWN* in order to *LEAP HIGHER*.

The most important thing to have as an asset is not money, gold, diamonds, cars, business, childred, religion, your body, or your looks; . . . the most important thing is your own mind. Using your mind wisely will improve your lifestyle and increase your life in added pleasurable years.

In Ft. Worth Texas a M.D. medical team, Carl Simonton and Stephanie Matthews Simonton, have been making news with their counseling and treatment of cancer patients. By treating the whole person using doses of chemotherapy, the treatment includes counseling and super nutrition methods with vitamin supplements. The theory is that the course of the disease can be reversed by reversing the personal attitudes that could start the disease. Patients admitted must be willing to consciously cooperate in changing their lives. Successes in the program have been reported in a number of publications.

Again Simonton's work demonstrates what holistic people believe: We give ourselves our illnesses. Not consciously, of course, but on a deeper level we are doing it ourselves. And, if we can make ourselves sick, why not use these same processes to make yourself well again, says Simonton.

Many people think that health is just the absence of disease. Rather it is a vital body process that releases the body's own healing powers. This state of well being is not inherited, or learned from other sources. To practice it includes taking the responsibility for our own health. The body's own healing power comes from (the logo above) the body, mind and spirit, in equilibrium. Spirit or phyche refers to a mysterious essential that combines the mental and physical.

To achieve this total well being requires some personal honesty with ourselves. This calls for changing some part of one's personal life style. It calls for embracing encouragement, not sequestering ourselves to change. Fears, hidden hates, frustration, all generate obvious action within our body as its own worst kind of mental stigma.

Nutrition awareness requires lots of study on our own, as well as guidance. Read but don't react, or look for health answers within "quick thinning diets or best sellers." Learn for yourself.

The second vital area is release of stress. This means to change your attitude as well as making use of advice on stress techniques. The basic mind idea in coping with stress is: the world isn't doing it to you. Its how you yourself react to the many outside conditions that are affecting you.

And third, we have dwelled on it somewhat, "to refresh the neural circuits. The greater sensing of our own totality.

Possibly you will feel this holistic health sounds too idealistic. But you have heard the "new Wave" of new feeling going on in this country. Really you are a lucky winner, to know what can be done for people today. In fact you have the ball (hint) all you need to do is run with it.

And lastly I am reminded that the human being is a very *complex organism*. We easily lose sight of our *very complex creation*. This biological symphony is orchestrated by our body, mind and spirit in harmonious changes.

But we think we can continue on "living" with multiple dissipations we discussed throughout this book. We even talk ourselves into believing anything but what we know to be the truth . . . but we are weak. We are too busy living a satisfying life we have become so used to, too busy to stop and pause for review. Too busy to remind ourselves we need to change our habits. Life seems too good to us, we are winners, so why worry about the future? . . . until the time comes for big health problems suddenly. Suffering and worry, large hospital and medical bills, mounting doctors expenses and drugs, . . . then it may be too late.

This describes closely the *self inflicted* 670,000 deaths on heart disease victims who will die in the next twelve months.

But thank the good Lord I am a lucky one, I know the problems. I can even joke about them. In closing, let's all look at the brighter side of life and think how lucky we really are. So cheer up, things could be worse. You could have given up plans to attend the Moscow Olympics in favor of a camping trip to Mount St. Helens.

EPILOG

Medicare is administered differently in different parts of the country. Various interpetitions of orders and bureaucratic wording sometimes open the door to a positive decision. Then there is the red tape.

In chapter 12, *Who needs Bypass Surgery?* There is noted important evidence. The National Institute of Health comment on bypass surgery. "That it is certainly doubtful that bypass surgery improves the function of the left venticular or that it makes the heart pump any better." This is evidence that $2 billion may be wasted on bypass surgery when it could have gone to a less costly and more positive therapy like chelation.

There is now under way an appeal and depending on the verdict there may be a class action suit initiated, by adding all cooperating patients who have been denied reimbursement. This complicated legal matter that will require decisions of attack after the legal decisions are rendered. Your chelation physician will keep you posted.

The Supreme Court will soon begin hearing an appeal instituted by the AMA the loser of a FTC suit for restraint of trade. This result could help decide the next legal action.

In summary, file a request for payment and an file an appeal for a fair hearing. Do not become frustrated or discouraged. Keep all records in duplicate good or bad, keep the door opened for any later acton that could result from political, legal or congressional actions.

DR. RAY EVERS . . . MARTYR FOR CHELATION THERAPY

Dr. Ray Evers is back in Alabama and has received financial backing to open the Sealy Springs Spa in Cottonwood, Alabama. Dr. Evers is in a struggle to recover financially from bankruptcy caused by so many legal battles with the government. He has made many positive inroads in a new successful health care clinic attached to the Spa. He needs to continue to render patient care he has done so successfully over the past thirty years.

Unfortunately he has again been handicapped by harrassment and conspiracy by local government authorities, prompted by unknown competitors. His medical enemies vow to "finish him off." We do not think this is possible knowing this strong willed religious man. He rolls with the punches beautifully considering all he has been through in the past 10 years, and as in the past we know he will come back stronger than ever. He is a fine example of high morality, intestinal fortitude and faith in God. And a fine unselfish physician also.

The charges against Dr. Evers followed a raid during his leading prayer services on a sunday morning January 25th. 1981. This was all part of an entrapment scheme, he says, to put him out of business on a felony charge that means loss of medical license in Alabama. The well publicized misinformation by the media caused a significant decrease in Dr. Ever's patient load and into the high prospective patient list turnover to keep a successful large operation on a paying basis.

Dr. Evers is continuing his good work while the long ordeal of appeal takes place.

Meanwhile through his international prominence he has been rewarded with a great honor and title of Sir Ray Evers. He has been knighted into the Ancient Order of the Knights of Malta, the oldest order of ancient chivalry headed by Queen Elizabeth II. His wife Marjorie was named a Dame in that order. They are the only Americans this year so honored in this order that dates back to the year 1048. It is composed of prominent physicians who are recognized for their humanitarian efforts.

In addition the Evers Health Center and Spa is being featured on the Christian Broadcasting Network and producers of the 700 Club. This two part documentary was recently filmed in Cottonwood. This is the largest independent satellite network with a potential audience of over 10 million people. It will feature Chelation Therapy and Dr. Evers help to thousands of hopeless victims and his legal episodes with conventional medicine and government.

Dr. Evers needs your support and your prayers.

Your contact: Evers Health Center, P.O. Box 587 Cottonwood, Ala. 36320. Telephone (205)691-2161

APPENDIX I

THE FACTS OF "LIFE".

It is not enough to have someone tell me to take an aspirin if I have a headache. To me it is more important to find out what is causing the headache than it is to find relief in some aspirin tablets. It is not enough to have someone suggest a vitamin tablet for a certain condition; it is important to know exactly why I should take the vitamin tablet. Remarks like "known to be protective" or "the benefits of the study show. . . ." or "suspect it acts as a. . . ." are not enough proof to suit my particular personality. I have learned that there is half-truth, truth, innuendo, or greed behind every statement I hear. If I did not find the cause of the headache I could become a chronic pill-taker, never finding out just what was wrong, just continuing to take aspirins as a habit each time my headache occurs.

Perhaps this is what's wrong with the medical profession and the habits the public are forced into. The doctor tells us what to do along with prescribing a drug. He treats the symptoms, not the cause. He just makes a diagnosis; the patient listens, possibly asks a few questions, picks up the prescription and pays his bill, all habit and conformity. Faith in the doctor and the prescription you acquire is really all you paid for, not to get well permanently.

We can blame this problem on habit; that's the way it's being done. Then there is hustle and bustle so common today, just not enough time for the doctor to explain fully (if he knows), nor the patient to have the time to "think" about some questions to ask the doctor. But really, you think, the prescription will take care of the problem; the doctor knows that. Possibly I can suggest that you should ask yourself, are you satisfied with the prescribed drug? Or would you like to take the time to get to the root of the problem and find a cure to that problem?

I never took an interest in vitamins before because almost everything I read left much information to be desired in the way of proof or facts pertaining to that particular vitamin's benefit. But as I read more and more I find out that it takes prolonged study and research in such a new scientific endeavor. The nutritional field is very young. Surely there are many studies, more new ones every day, and slowly conclusions are published. It is only a great many conclusions all the same that leads professionals to mention proof of studies. So I would rather rely on a reliable source of information rather than "hearsay" that is so easy to find today. I like to see wording such as, "The need in human nutrition is recognized or has been established, etc.". And I would feel more comfortable hearing it from a professional physician who specialized in nutrition.

So here starts our review. Cells are microscopic structures of four main types (the four are not important) but the cells are organized into tissues, tissues into organs, organs into systems, and systems into the final unit. . . . the body.

SURVIVAL is one of the functions of the body. Homeostasis, metabolism, and integration are some of the complex components necessary for survival.

HOMEOSTASIS. Imagine a swimming pool with five feet of water in it, with water running in one side and running out the other side, but staying level at almost five feet. This is an example of dynamic equilibrium, the characteristic of homeostasis. That water level is important to the body also; health and survival depend upon the body maintaining or quickly restoring homeostasis. When we perspire a great deal we become thirsty; our body tells us to drink more water to maintain homeostasis.

METABOLISM. This is another of the great works of the body and survival; chemical change is a simple meaning. Metabolism consists of chemical reactions going on inside living cells, a function made up of other functions. Such functions as ingestion, digestion, absorption of food, respiration, circulation, anabolism, catabolism, secretion, excretion, and even "control" of these many processes.

INTEGRATION. This means unification. To achieve intergration of so many functions, nerve impulses and chemicals control the sequences and the extent of bodily activities. Chief among these control chemicals are enzymes, vitamins and hormones. Death releases matter from this unifying control, and the material of the body moves again toward *dis*integration. . .life is organization, death is disintegration; illness is in between.

PROTOPLASM IS LIVING MATTER. All cells, whether plant cells or animal cells, are composed of protoplasm, the "*physical basis of life.*" The main elements of protoplasm are oxygen, nitrogen, carbon and hydrogen. These and other elements are combined to form various compounds, mainly proteins, carbohydrates, lipids (fats and fat-like compounds) and inorganic salts. These and other elements are combined to form various compounds of which WATER is, by far, the most abundant. Various cells contain elements of human protoplasm. Here is a chart of the percentages contained within the cell:

ELEMENTS	PERCENT	COMPOUND	PERCENT
Oxygen	65	Water	75
Carbon	18	Proteins	20
Nitrogen	3	Lipids	2
Hydrogen	10	Inorganic Salts	1
Calcium	2	Carbohydrates	2
Phosphorus	1		
Potassium	0.35		
Sulfur	0.25		
Chlorine	0.15		
Chlorine	0.15		
Sodium	0.15		
Magnesium	0.05		
Iron	0.004		
Others	0.046		

If you weigh 100 pounds, your body has in it the various substances shown above. The cells in the body cannot do work without the substances listed. Cells are made up of four basic elements: Carbon (C); Oxygen (0); Hydrogen (H); and Nitrogen (N). The balance of elements are necessary but in much smaller amounts.

The four basic elements (C, H, O, N) and the others can be gotten **only** from the food we eat, from the water and other liquids you drink, and from the air you breathe. These substances are used as nutrition for the body.

Carbohydrates are made up of carbon, hydrogen and oxygen, as the make-up of the word indicates. Sugar and starch is the make-up . . . pies, cake, bread, candy, etc. They are oxidized in the body . . . yielding energy for the work of the cells.

Proteins contain the same elements plus (N) nitrogen, and used by the body of growth of the tissues. **Fats** have the same elements as carbohydrates but the amount of hydrogen is greater . . . used for energy. **Water** is needed to dissolve foods. Unless they are first dissolved, they cannot be used by the body. As you breathe, you oxidize the chemical energy in the nutrients to be used by the body cells.

Not a single cell in the body can live more than a few minutes without oxygen. Every heart cell must have food and oxygen. Every cell produces waste which must be removed. Life-sustaining then means oxygen, energy, and waste excretion in the body processes.

The cell is the smallest unit of living matter that contains an independent existence and reproduces itself. Cells are the simplest structural units of the body, but even their complexity taxes the imagination. The cell is a functional as well as a structural unit. Each cell carries on functions that characterize it as "alive" and, in addition, performs some special function for the body as a whole, such as secretion by epithelial cells, contraction by muscle cells, transmission by nerve cells, etc.

Each cell, in other words, fulfills its own requisites for life and in addition, also contributes to the life of the entire body. If it was not for this great power of self-renewal we would be dead long ago. And vice versa; the body performs functions of each of its parts. It supplies them with nutrients and oxygen and removes their wastes. In short, a relationship of mutual interdependence exists between the body as a whole and each of its various parts. Optimum health of the body depends upon optimum health of each of its parts down to even the smallest cell. This is where we must "look" when we think of our individual health maintenance. And of course, it is better to look for natural means of attaining health. Conventional medicine treats our health with drugs that can result in artificial reactions and temporary relief. The new wave of medical men uses natural means for relief of illness, so the results are more permanent and positive.

Many people think about food the same way they think about gasoline for their cars. . .that is, just put more in as it depletes itself.

While food is fuel for the body, it is needed to replace cells that are dying or worn out. While we can call food fuel, it is more accurate to call it "energy."

While energy comes from the food we eat, it is important to know "how it works". The smallest amount of energy we are concerned with here is an "anion" a negative ion which is an alkaline substance. A "cation" is a positive ion, and an acid substance. The cation has more energy than an anion. These forces meet against each other (resistance) and create the proper balance between anions and cations that produce energy.

If a person gets sick there are not enough anionic substances present to supply the energy needs from the cationic substances eaten, so you can call it improper digeston.

The liver can manufacture these molecules of anionic substances into extremely large numbers of different *enzymes*. The proper balance of the enzymes is part of the nutrition picture.

In order to move about and reproduce, living things must capture energy. Plants do by the sun's energy and store it as chemical energy. Animals must capture their energy supply by feeding on other living things, or things that were once alive. The capture of energy is another characteristic of all living things. . . another life activity.

The captured energy is released by oxidation. In oxidation, the living thing generally uses oxygen for the activities of the cell. The energy released by oxidation of food substances in the cell is not known, but is used by the cells in what may be called the cell energy process.

Nutrition is a characteristic of living things. Nutrition furnished the energy for the cell to reproduce, and for the growth and repair of tissues.

A living thing is an organism. It is organized in a very special way to perform life-activities. . .to grow, to reproduce, to respire, and to get its store of energy which is food substance.

You are an organism; you are alive; you need a special environment in which to carry on life's activities.

An enormous amount of digestive enzymes are secreted by the human digestive tract each day. The average adult's daily secretion comes to more than 2 gallons.

Salivary secretion.....mouth.....	6 cups
Gastric secretion.....stomach.....	10 cups
Bile.....liver......................	2 cups
Pancreatic juice.................	3 cups
Intestional mucus secretion......	12 cups
Total..................	33 cups

As there Is nothing more precious than good health, we need the best food obtainable for these juices to act upon. Good nutrition depends on these juices, just as these juices depend on good food. Here lies a major problem causing illness. . .artifically processed foods.

Other factors, of course enter into the picture and help the good work of these enzymes. One is to be cheerful as we eat, because the condition of our mind does have an effect on the the secreton of juices as well as the digestion of food. The person with a calm mind while he eats is allowing his digestive tract to function normally.

Good tasting foods that are attractive in appearance and served in a pleasing atmosphere help free secretion and make for good digestion. Basic to this process of digestion is a good, pleasing, non-processed food. Only food quality determines this.

Mother Nature has given our digestive tract great automatic functioning. We can profit from the enzyme function of normal digestion without entirely understanding it.

We could starve if our body chemistry could not convert protein into human amino acids needed for the heart, arteries, muscles and glands; and if it could not change all food into the subsistence for life itself.

The enzymes in your body and the enzymes in the food work together to increase the efficiency of the heart and the arterial system. All life processes such as breathing, moving around, digestion, growing up, are all controlled by enzyme activity.

An enzyme in your saliva converts the starch of bread into sugar. Enzymes in your stomach and intestines break down proteins into the simpler building blocks of amino acids. The enzymes digest starches, sugars, and fats. Wherever the enzymes are, they are there to speed up chemical changes in the body.

All food enzymes are destroyed at about 25 degrees Fahrenheit above blood temperature. As enzymes and the vitamins in foods begin to disappear at cooking temperatures above 123 degrees F, it is readily apparent that nutritional losses are brought about by long cooking.

Despite the complexity of the body organism, the individual components must play a specific part in a mighty biochemical symphony, all in tune with each other if health is to be maintained. This concept of wholeness is sometimes referred to as "holistic health."

OUT OF ALL THE FOOD NUTRIENTS OUR CELLS RECEIVE, THEY MANUFACTURE ONLY ONE THING. . . . LIFE.

Knowing all this biological information and much more about this complex body of ours, it seems quite simple to maintain good health. All we have to do is know what to eat, how and where to live, and how to lead a happy life so we can stay healthy.

But meanwhile, we disrupt all this wellness by our illness and disease. And it no longer is simple anymore as we try to restore the original life process again. In fact, it has become a universal puzzle. We have not learned completely how to reverse this biological chemical process. . .we have some answers and we keep trying.

I am a lucky living convert from this disruptive process and disease. I believe now it is easier to prevent the problem than it is to try and reverse it.

APPENDIX II

THE AGING PUZZLE

The puzzle of life! The how long we are going to live theory is changing. They speak now of how much longer we are going to live. Science knows a great deal more about how to extend life, than what we are lead to believe. We could even suspect because of the wealth of research already, and the FDA problem, that information is not being doled out to us. Then too, the government needs many answers on how to cope with extended life in this inflationary age.

Its not all the old thinking anymore of, be born, grow up, reproduce, and gradually fade out of the picture. Now there's many researchers involved and there's nature's own work, and the drug industry. But there is a lot "betwix't and between."

There is a biological clock for the human being and well as plant life. The extension of that clock is the name of the game. One area of new attention is genetic engineering. They are now producing laboratory genes that can do many miraculous things for cell growth, by gene change, for improved life both for animal, plants and man.

There are FREE RADICALS that are becoming better understood and their defense is becoming perfected. Dr. Denham Harman, of the University of Nebraska, advanced the early popular theory of "free radicals." Research continues that is also associated with the origin of disease.

There appears certain molecules in our bodies that get disarranged. Their electronic components are effected by cosmic rays, the sun, or other enviromental factors.

The radicals, a free electron, is a negative charge that has the desire to be attached to a working system with a positive charge, like a magnet. But areas of our body do *NOT* want to be affected by these wandering radical electrons. Although certain abnormal systems or organs such as cancer cells will accept them. Those that scavenger deadly deposits, accept them and are affected by them.

This unwelcome union of activity just compounds the problem or the injury to the cells and tissues, which try to maintain normal activity and existance. The extreme activity increases as the tendency to capture more electrons grows. But in time these free electrons do damage to the body, effecting metabolism, decreasing cell proliferation or aging the cell. As the parts of the molecules combine and grow, so does these free radicals, causing havoc that is associated with so many causes of disease. Free radical reactions generally start chain reactions that multiply so fast it can effect thousands more reactions.

Free radicals can now be detected by scientific tests by determination of the unpaired electron.

We have already mentioned in early chapters Vitamin E as an antioxidant in the method to attack this problem. Vitamin E has been found to extend cell life by prolonging life past the normal 50 generations, and up to 200 generations in animal studies. To normal cells this means we can gradually alter our body chemistry with vitamin E.

Another theory is by Dr. Hans Selye, Physicologist at the University of Montreal. Dr. Selye is world famous for his research with stress. He says that stress is an important causative factor in the aging process. It is said that stress is the tearing down of man's body and mind. Dr. Selye has said that part of the problem lies with lack of vitamin E also.

These are the main hypothesis; there are many more you will hear about in the future. But like any research in medicine not all the theories prove successful or not all are generally accepted. It is a constant fight to gain recognition from any research as there are many opposing views. It really has to be won the hard way by the individual's own persistance.

GEROVITAL H3 OR GH3

One of the publicized events in this Country concerns the approval by the FDA of Gerovital H3 or GH3. This is a drug that is believed to be the key to rejuvenation, an antidepressant that may make cells reproduce longer.

It is the facinating story of the discovery by Dr. Anna Aslan of Romania. Of the much publicized and thorough testing of the drug in this Country and the ultimate adamant stand against approval of the drug by the FDA.

The drug Gerovital H3 or GH3 has been called *"the fountain of youth."* Studies in Europe and America have been going on for thirty years. Over 200,000 people have used GH3 already. It is approved for use in Romania, England, France, Italy and Switzerland.

If you are wealthy you could go to Romania for treatments like the Gabor sisters, Mao Zedung, Ho Chi Minh and Kirk Douglas has done.

Then there is the similiarity of GH3 to a drug that has been used in this Country successfully for over thirty years. The drug is procaine, better known as novacaine. In addition there is a link in GH3 with a well known medical drug called MOA or monoamine oxidase, an enzyme. MOA has been well known in medical circles as a drug that could cure depression, and slow down the aging process. What was needed for its sucess and use was an inhibitor so there would be no detrimental side effects. It finally turned out that MOA combined with procaine was the key to Dr. Aslan's discovery.

But despite the millions of older people helped all over Europe, despite the elaborate testing done in this Country, the FDA remained adamant in determining proof was not adequate that GH3 was an anti-depressant drug.

Dr. Aslan believes that the body's inherent natural ability to replace cells lost through disease and age diminishes through the years. GH3 supplements the body's ability to regenerate new cells. She is convinced that cell regeneration is responsible for the return of youthfullness in older people.

Without allowing the reader to believe this writer is being carried away by the overwhelming evidence in support of GH3. While the evidence in Europe is not accepted by the FDA; the insurmountable restrictions placed in the standards of testing by the FDA on GH3, there is a similiarity in the problem with EDTA and the FDA.

DMSO—TOMMORROW'S ASPIRIN?

Another well known and much publicized drug is DMSO or Dimethyl-suloxide. The plot to the story is similiar to

GH3. The conclusion of the testing procedures is similiar as is the rewards for the drugs use.

The story reads like a science fiction thriller as it was reported by Pat McGrady Sr. in THE PERSECUTED DRUG. THE STORY OF DMSO. (CHARTER) It is the complete reporting on DMSO its history and the endless effort of Dr. Stanley Jacob of the University of Oregon, against the power of the FDA and the AMA.

Without a question of doubt this is truly a wonder drug as future experience will no doubt reveal. Not so much as a reliever of pain but as a quick transporter of other drugs to affected parts of the body.

DMSO has beneficial ability, depending on its concentration in use and if applied topically or intravenously. From acute bursitis, low back pain, rhumatoid arthritis to ichemic and varicose ulcers, plebitis, gout all the way to acne and psoriasis.

DMSO like EDTA has power to chelate certain minerals out of molecules that has application in lead poisoning and related disorders. DMSO has the power to dissolve body chemicals such as fatty acids, steroids and polysaccarides. It gets rid of the water shell around many substances and then dissolves them; that is, it floods the space between the solute molecules, delicately separating and suspending them.

DMSO denatures or demolishes the basic chemical components of life, neuleic acids and some proteins; it breaks them up so they never can be put together again. In low concentrations DMSO may gently dissolve some proteins and activate them. This dual influence on proteins endows DMSO with a vast potential of enzyme effects. Enzymes are proteins which catalyze in many hundreds of reactions in the body's essential chemistry. By activating or inhibiting various enzyme systems, DMSO turns on and off various physical and mental functions. This is only the start of its applications.

In addition, the drug can make antibiotic-resistant bacteria more sensitive to antibiotics again. DMSO attacks the disease itself, rather than just the symptoms. This kills bacteria and prevents their growth and could do the same thing for viruses and fungi.

There have been six different resolutions already introduced into Congress so that the FDA or the Congress can expedite the approval of this drug. The whole idea is to relieve the FDA of its power over the American people.

Many of the preventative medicine societys' members have made inroads in the cure or relief of the pain of cancer. Their metabolic therapy has included a therapeutic approach to malignancy. They base it on the premise that cancer is the sign of a chronic metabolic disfunction. And after performing all the tests mentioned in an earlier chapter, DMSO cancer therapy is started. The intravenous solution is monitored very closely for signs of toxicity. Patients receive Vitamin C, laetrile, and DMSO in various concentrations. Pain is relieved and the self-healing therapy commences. When their immunological defenses are restored, a patient is said to feel positive signs of regression. The patients own positive attitude and cooperation is needed for this turn-around healing process. We hear many reports of positive help from metabolic and therapeutic therapy. In fact there are no serious side effects in this therapy as we see so often with chemotherapy used by conventional medicine.

Now to the two question you would surely ask. Is DMSO safe? Under most conditions as applied by a physician with the medically made specifications, it is safe. As applied by the average person and purchased as a commercial solvent it is doubtful in the handling how safe it could be. Cleanliness and caution is advised.

What about approval by the government? Here again the same story of the FDA's controlled study demands or double blind studies. This is where the FDA and conventional medicine "hang their hats" on their righteous stand, behind the law. But this is impossible in the case of DMSO as the patient tastes the drug very quickly and the garlic odor is the clue that there cannot be a placebo.

There have been thousands of bottles of commercial DMSO sold to thousands of people with varying problems of health, I have heard of no problems of misuse or tragedies with this DMSO. I can assure you that if there were any problems or scandal with all the widespread use, the headlines would be screaming the bad news. Instead we see interviews on TV about DMSO as well as newpaper reports that would surely indicate any problems, if there were any. So how safe is safe?

In 1979 the FDA approved DMSO after a struggle that lasted more than ten years, for the treatment of interstitial cystitis, a bladder ailment. This leaves you with a feeling that what is good for one ailment should be good for other ailments particularly when administered in the exact same way. But with the power of the FDA to determine safety and efficacy for any ailment at all, the argument is lost in the power handed to them by the Congress.

The bottom line is we have various new methods that help reverse the aging process. We have oppressive problems that prevent the administration of the various methods that should help all of us. But we have hope that the future will be very good to us in extending our lives for better living with less suffering. How it all turns out is up to the *effort of each of us.*

APPENDIX III

COMPARISONS INDICATE HELP IS NEEDED.

Few of up stop to realize that we have been risking our very existence for centuries. The risks to us are the same as with the animal or insect and really it is for survival. We still have earthquakes, floods, accidents, hurricanes and fires. As our population exploded and new advances took hold, we have pesticides, additives, birth control pills, contaminated water, and animal fattners just to name a few of our newly developed hazards.

Despite these everyday risks the population is still growing. Our birth rate, by design, is declining as young people find it difficult to cope with the new problems of the world. Accordingly, our way of life is changing. Our health costs are rising and we are affected by social and medical problems that seem out of our reach for our solutions.

Some of the problems are:

The government continues to establish new laws to protect us. Even though the government is not our keeper or protector it seems politically feasable. But we must pay for these services provided by government and the cost is getting out of hand.

The power of conventional medicine influences government and our very lives. They say have faith in them, trust them. Of course this has been proven wrong as our false hopes and health care costs are nearing strangulation status. Millions of sick people are barely living in a life of misery and pain, and don't know they can be helped back to health by other means.

It appears that the United States is out to top all records among Nations of the World with the highest cost health care of all. We are second in per capita death rate in the world also. How much of this can we stand.

Our 252 billion dollar yearly health care bill is not only staggering but shameful. We see the results in every hospital, rest home, mental institution, school for the retarded, jails and cemetaries.

The protectionism Frankenstein that we all helped to create is about to devour us with death, suffering and fiscal bankrupcy. It seems so unnecessary as it is taking freedom away from all of us.

This writer believes it is high time we all took responsibility for our own health and destiny. Just as terminal cancer patients accept responsibility for their condition and learn to heal themselves in cooperation with a knowledgable physician; so too should all of us start to think for themselves rather than relying on government. It is being done every day by thousands of people. Just look at the business the health food stores are doing. Look at the new patients that are going to the modern preventive medicine physicians. These physicians are winning new patients every day.

There are many problems that need resolving such as:

- **The influence of the AMA on government must be throttled.**
- **The guidelines of the FDA need to be changed.**
- **Americans need a law to allow them FREEDOM OF MEDICAL CHOICE.**

The pages of this book featured the ability of EDTA and chelation therapy to help all people out of problems of the heart and circulatory system. There has been two of many drugs reported, GH3 and DMSO, that could possibly help old people and many already afflicted with disease. And we have emphasized the new breed of modern physician that can help all the people.

Here's what these three drugs and their therapies can do for us:

- *Retarding the aging process, including memory loss, vitality and energy. Retirement time can be posponed in years,*
- *Benefit: easing Social Security drains and the tax burden on younger people.*
- *Reversing occlusive artery disease, angina pain and other circulatory problems.*
- *Benefit: Free the government and its people from the high cost of surgery, suffering and death.*
- *Relieve pain of injury and accident and of the crippling diseases.*
- *Benefits: less drain on absenteeism and inactivity that leads to general health decline and disability.*
- *Relief of the problems of the nervous system, such as migraine, visual, hearing and mental problems.*
- *Benefit: Less drain on mental hospitals, crime and old age deficiencies.*

HEALTH CARE PROBLEMS COMPRISING ABOUT 80 PERCENT OF OUR HEALTH CARE COSTS.

DIRECTLY OR INDIRECTLY HELPED BY THREE DRUGS

Note: All drugs and their therapies appear safe and non-habit forming when used by a licensed physician. Patient health improved wholly or in part.

EDTA CHELATION THERAPY. * Intravenous.	GEROVITAL H3 or GH3 * Intravenous or tablet	DMSO * Topical or intravenous
Occlusive artery disease	angina pain	athletic injury
stroke	menapaulas syndrome	angina pain
angina pain	hypertension	eschemic & varicose ulcer
hypertension	diabetes	lead poisoning
diabetes	arthritis	diabetes
arthritis	schizophrenia	arthritis
schizophrenia	memory loss	schizophrenia
senility	scheroderma	mental retardation
muscular distrophy	multiple sclerosis	scleroderma
gangrene	moody life	acne/psoriasis
claudication	muscular waste	gangrene
digitalis toxicity	insomnia	plebitis, gout, sprians
necrotic ulcers	gastrointestinal ulcer	sinusitus
lead/metal poisoning	depression	burns/sunburn
kidney stones	sexual impotence	rhumatism
heart calcification	vision problems	nerve blindness
*possible burning at the infusion site corrected by drip adjustment.	*requires skin test for allergic reaction.	*possible itching, burning, drying skin, sunburn-like effect. Rare hypersen-sitivity reaction.

Note: Cancer in its various forms was purposely omitted from the above lists. Some cancers have been helped by these drugs used in conjunction with other drugs and/or vitamin and mineral supplementation.

Some of the scientific experiments and testing on these drugs for their usefullness has been completed. Any future experience and experimental work will enhance the drugs use and possible add new usefullness for all.

But please dear reader, do not believe that GH3, DMSO and EDTA are cure alls. Most of the evidence on GH3 and DMSO have been ignored by the FDA. Research progressed awhile, then stopped. I do not mean to mislead anyone with such a long list. These substances are not the ultimate answers possible, but evidence indicates that if given a chance to use these substances, past research will be vindicated and eventually prove to change our lives for the better.

APPENDIX IV

GRANOLA CEREALS UPDATE

In the chapter on nutrition I mentioned granola and cereals, then later I mentioned mixing the store bought granola's to my wife's ready-to-eat cereal. Citing the delicious taste and the stomach-filling nature of granola I overlooked the unwanted ingredients that are so hard to eliminate from any store-bought food.

Now I see these ready-made cereals have sugar and saturated fats in large amounts. While these fats and sugars may make the cereal more filling; the milk added makes the absorption and expansion really the main reason for its filling nature.

But whether we mix the granola into our recommended recipe or, add a supermarket brand of granola in combination, we are inviting problems with unwanted ingredients. Here's why:

> They contain little or no bran and usually a small amount of salt. We receive large amounts of saturated fats (the worst kind) The sweet taste is still there in white sugar, brown sugar or honey which are all empty calories.

This is the nutritional picture of granola cereals found in the supermarket. Post Cereals plain or raisin; 100% Natural, plain or raisins and dates; Heartland with coconut or raisins.

Analyzing one cereal, the 100% Natural, we find 130 caloies in one ounce or 1/3 cup dry; 17 gm carbohydrate, 8gm sugar; 3gm protein, and fat 4 gm. 80% of the fat is saturated and 20% is mono or poly unsaturated.

As we see in most all processed foods the manufacturer cannot get away from hydrogenated fats that harden inside of us. Adding fruits in our recipe together with those sweets added by the manufacturer makes the cereal possibly too sweet but palatable. So you see granola bought in the store isn't the best answer to fats and calories.

The question is how can we make this cereal better? How can we make it more nutritious, with less fats and sugars so it is still delicious food? The answer is simple, just make your own.

Here is the basic part of granola cereal. After the basics you may add anything you like. The need in the recipe is to make the cereal crunchy and eye-appealing. In order to do so we need to add water and oil so that in the baking we don't end up making it unattractive and burnt to a crisp. This makes the cereal easier to chew and more palatable.

5 cups rolled oats
1 cup water

1/4 cup honey
1/2 teaspoon cinnamon
1 cup bran

1/2 cup sunflower seeds raw*
1/2 cup wheat germ raw*
1 teaspoon lecithin liquid.
*If raw items are unavailable, leave them out and add toasted items AFTER cooling the batch

Mix all ingredients well until all are thourougly moistened. Spread out on a cookie sheet and bake in a preheated oven at 250 deg. F. Stirring often is essential. When the steam stops escaping the batch is finished. It takes about 45 minutes When cooled completely add raisins or other dried fruits and the (*) dry ingredients. Be sure to substitute water for honey if less sweetness is desired.

There is about 87 calories in one ounce or 1/3 cup serving. Remember there is sweetness and calories in raisins and dates. Fresh fruit added for variety can also replace the need for sweetness.

Try it, I am sure you will like it. Its more filling, has the needed bran for proper assimilation in the stomach and relief of constipation, less calories and fat and good for you.

In this new recipe we have cut down on saturated fats and sugar. Most all the sweetness can be optional and added to each bowl-full as it is served. Adding any fresh or dried fruit can add to the variety as the need arises. But remember with such variety we add calories. And do not be carried away with large portions.

RECOMMENDED READING AND BILIOGRAPHY

AAMP: The American Academy of Medical Preventics, 8383 Wilshire Blvd., Beverly Hills, CA

ALSLEBEN, Rudolph, & Shute, Wilfred; *How To Survive New Health Catastrophies,* Survival Publications, Anaheim, CA 1973

ANTHONY, Catherine Parker; *Textbook Of Anatomy & Physiology,* C.V. Mosby Co. 21-27, 557-559

BAILEY, Herbert; GH3 Will It Keep Our Younger Younger? Bantom Books 1977

BERKO, Robert; Special Chiropractic issue *Caveat Emptor Bulletin* 4-11, 21-23, 2-4

BERKO, Robert; *Oversupply Of Doctors Should Bring End Of Medical School Subsidies,* Cavest Emptor Bulletin 12/80, 2

BLACK, David; *Medicine And The Mind.* Playboy Magazine 4/80, 79

BOYD, Ronald; *The Shattering Effects Of An Emotional Killer: Stress* St. Petersburg Times 9/18/80

BUSINESS WEEK; *"Drive To Extend Patients"* 2/16/81

BRODY, Jane E.; *Risks Seen In Type A Behavior;* N.Y. Times reprint St. Petersburg Times 10/22/80

BURKITT, Dennis & Painter, N.S.; *Digestive Disease* Vol. 19 1974 9864

BURKETT, Dennis; *The Evidence Leavons: We Invite Colon Cancer;* Medical World News 8/11/72

CALCIUM CHELATION OF ATHEROSCLEROSIS: NINE YEARS OF CLINICAL EXPERIENCE; 14th Annual Meeting American College of Angiology 1968

CHELATION THERAPY OF OCCLUSIVE ARTERIOSCLEROSIS IN DIABETIC PATIENT; Angiology 15 1964 379

CLARKE, N.E. & Clarke C.N.; *Treatment Of Angina Pectoris With EDTA* Am Jr Med Sci 1956 656-666

CHERASKIN, E., Ringsdorph, W.M.; *Phychodietetichs* Stein and Day 1975

CARBERRY, James; *Physicians Can Detect Clues That Indicate Chance Of Illness* 11/8/72

CARPENTER, Donald G.; *Chelation Therapy's Correction To Biological Aging* Rejuvination Magazine 6/29 1980

CASDORPH, Richard H.; *EDTA Chelation Therapy 11 Efficacy In Brain Disorders* Journel of Holistic Medicine, Fall 1981. Human Sciences Press

CHALMERS, Thomas C., Stern Alfred R.; *The Staggering Cost Of Prolonging Life* Business Week 2/23/81 19-20

CHARASKIN, E. Ringsdorph W.M.; *Predictive Medicine;* Exposition Press N.Y.

CLEVE, T.L.; *The Saccharine Disease* vol. 19, Bristol, 1974

CLEVE, T.L.; *Peptic Ulcer,* Wright, 1962

CHARASKIN, E. Ringsdorph W.M.; *New Hope For Incurable Diseases,* Arco, 1971

COE, Marion; *Patient, Heal Thyself* St. Petersburg Times Floridian Section 7/20/80

COHN, Victor; *Quit Big Business Medicine, Doctors Told,* St. Petersburg Times/Wash. Post 10/23/80

COOPER, Kennith H.; *The New Aerobics,* Bantom Books & Evans 1968

CRANTON, Elmer M.; *Hair Nutrition Analysis In Preventive Medicine, IFPM,* Annandale, VA

DALLY, A.G.; *Readers Guide To Modern Medicine,* Signet, 1969

DAVIS, Adelle; *Lets Eat Right To Keep Fit,* Jove HBC

DE BACKY, Michael, Debachy, Lois; *Prescription For Disaster,* Readers Digest, 12/80

DEMBART, Lee; *Genetic Engineering,* St. Petersburg Times 1/18/81

DUMONT, Belinda; *Orthohealing,* Omni Mag. 2/80

FRIEDMAN, Myer & Rosenman; *Type A Behavior For Your Heart,* Knopf, Annuals of Research, 1974

GOLDWAG, William H.; *Chelation Therapy; Taking A Hint From Nature* Patient reprint AAMP Library

GORDON, Garry F.; *Hair Analysis, Its Uses And Limitations,* Reprint Lets Live Magazine 11/80

GORDON, F. Kannel, W.B., Sorlie P.P.; *The Framingham Study ,* National Institute of Health 1971

GUTTING, Robert D.; *Chelation Therapy: A Short Course On Description, Use & Function,* Tec Pub., Topkea, KA

GREENBERG, Daniel S.; *Can We Prevent The M.D.'s Surplus From Pushing Up The Cost Of Medical Care?* Caveat Emptor Bulletin 6/80 10

GORDON, Garry F.; *History And Mechanisms Of Action Of EDTA Chelation Therapy,* Reprint from NAPM vol. 1, 11-20

GRUMBLES Lloyd, Lutz Howard; Interview, Washington D.C. from Speech at AAMP Seminar 1980

GREENSPAN, Emily; *Your Hairdresser, The Nutritionist,* Self Mag. 8/80 46-48

GORDON, Garry F., Vance, Robert B.; *EDTA For Arteriosclerosis: History And Mechanisms Of Action,* Osteopathic Annuals 4:38-62 2/76

HOFFER, Abrams, Osmond, Humphrey; *How To Live With Schizophrenia,* University 66

HALSTEAD, Bruce; *Results Of Cerebral Blood Flow Study After EDTA Chelation Therapy Talk AAMP,* Seminar, 1979

HALSTEAD, Bruce; *Chelation Therapy Patients Handbook,* Golden Quill Colton Ca 1978

HARPER, Harold, Culbert, Michael L., *Mans Miracle Molecule,* Reprinted from *How To Beat The Killer Diseases,* Arlington House 1977

JACOBSON, Michael; *Diet And Health: A Missing Link In Your Doctors Education,* Caveat Emptor Bulletin 7/80

KUMMERLOW, Fred, Kasmaii, Meena, Burnside Laboratory Univ of Illinois Urbana *Study On Eggbeaters,* Pediatrics Vol. 53 #4 4/74

KELL, George F.; *Brief Filed With Curtis Klahs* in matter of Ophelia Clementino 10/9/76

KELL, George F.; *Decision Of The Hearing Officer* Occidenital Life Insurance Co. Ca. Proceedings 10/13/76 HIC 236-03-7068-13

KITCHELL, J.R., Metzer, L & Seven, M.J.; *Potential Uses Of Chelation Therapy In Treatment Of Cardiovascular Disease* 19:798, 1961

HOCHMAN, Gloria; *The Bypass Question,* Today Mag. 8/5/79

HARLAND, Barbara; *Grandma Called It Roughage,* FDA Consumer 1977

HOLDERBY, W.W.; *Chelation Therapy,* reprint from Natural Food and Farming Vol. 26 #1 6/79

HUSTON, Philip; *Seven Common Operations We May No Longer Need,* Next Mag. 10/80 70-73

KOENIG, Albert; *Surgery Rate Rising Faster Than Population,* St. Petersburg Times, 7/4/80

KUGLER, Hans; *Slowing Down The Aging Process,* Pyramid, 1973

LAUGHLIN, John; *Ninty Days To A Better Heart,* Arco 58, 148-151

LEAHEY, Patrick, Sen. (D) *Diet And Health A Missing Link In Doctors Education,* Caveat Emptor Bulletin 8/80

MUELLER, William Behr, *Is It Really Necessary,* Reprint from Bestways 10/77

MATCHAN, Don; *Heart, Stroke Victims Turn To Chelation Therapy And Are Glad,* National Health Federation Bulletin 2/80 Now called "Public Scrutiny."

MALTZ, Maxwell; phycho Cybernetics. Simon & Shuster

MENDELSHON, Robert; *Confessions Of A Medical Heretic,* Warner 1979

MIKITINA, E.K. et al; *Treatment Of Arteriosclerosis With Trilon B* (EDTA) Kardiologia 72, 37

McCAMY, John C. & Priestly, James; *Human Life Styling,* Harper & Row 1977

McGRADY, Patrick Sr.; *DMSO The Persecuted Drug,* Charter, Gossett & Dunlop

MURRAY, Frank, Adams, Ruth; *Vitamin E Wonder Worker Of The 70's* Larchmont 71

MENDELSHON, Robert; *Try Chropractic,* Caveat Emptor Bulletin 2/80

MACY Foundation; *Biologic Reactions Of Chelating Agents,* Fifth Conference on Metabolic Interrelations. 54, 344-358

MILLMAN, Marcia; *The Unkindest Cut,* reprint from New West adapted before publication William Morrow, 1977

NEW YORK TIMES; *Scientists Studing Packets Of Longevity, Hope That The Aging Process Can Be Understood And Controlled.* 2/11/73

NULL, Garry, *The GH3 Controversy,* Caveat Emptor Bulletin 8/80

PASSWATER, Richard; *Supernutrition For Healthy Hearts,* Jove 1978

PASSWATER, Richard; *SUPERNUTRITION The Megavitamin Revolution,* Pocket Books 1976

PASSWATER, Richard; *The Easy No-Flab Diet,* Richard Marek, 1981

PUBLIC SCRUTINY MAGAZINE, Of the National Health Federation Monrovia Calif 91016

PROXMIRE, William, Sen (D) *You Can Do It . . . Diet And Exercise Plan,* Simon & Shuster 1973

PAULING, Linus; *Vitamin C And The Common Cold,* Pyramid 1977

SCHAUSS, A.; *Diet, Crime And Deliquency,* Parker House 1980

SCHRODER, Henry A.; *Geological Survey Of City Water Supplies Covering 90• Of Metropolitian Population And 58• Of U.S. Population,* 1050-51

SCHUTE, Wilfred E.; *Vitamin E For Ailing And Healthy Hearts,* Pyramid, 1977

SHOCK, Nathan; National Institute of Health, Geronotology Research Center, University of Maryland

SIEGAL, Sanford, *Dr. Segals Natural Fiber Permanent Weight Loss Diet,* Dell 1975

SIMONTON, Carl & Simonton, Stephanie Matthews, Counciling Cancer and Research Center, Ft. Worth, TX

STONE, Irwin J.; *The Healing Factor Of Vitamin E Against Disease,* Grosset & Dunlop 1972

WILLIAMS, Roger J.; *Nutrition Against Diseases: Environmental Protection,* Pitman 1971

WRIGHT, James; *The Sweet Taste Of Success,* Caveat Emptor Bulletin 6/79

TOWARD HEALTH DIETS, U.S. Food and Nutrition Board 5/27/80

TUSNET, Leonard, *The Medicine Men,* St. Martins Press and reprinted and available from Caveat Emptor Bulletin 620 Fr, Freeman St. Orange, N.J. 07050

VOICE OF MEDICAL FREEDOM, Monthly, Westlake Village CA 91359

GLOSSARY OF MEDICAL TERMS

ACCRETION. Adhearance of parts normally separated...accumulation.
ANEURYISM. A localized dialation of a blood vessel, usually an artery wall.
ANGIOGRAPHY. Radiographic recording of contrast material injected into arteries.
ARTHERIOSCLEROSIS. Thickening or hardening of the arteries.
ATROPHY. Decrease in size of a normally developed organ or tissue.
ARTERIOLE. Small arteries
APOPLEXY. A stroke caused by a cerebral hemorrage or bloking of a blood vessel.
BLOOD UREA CONCENTRATION. Urea overstimulates the heart causing tension & restlessness.
BLOOD CLOT. A plug that normally forms when a vessel is injured or weakened.
CALCIFICATION. Deposits of lime salts in tissue and bones.
CAPILLARIES. Minute blood vessels.
CARBOHYDRATE. The scientific name for sugars, starches and cellulose.
CARCINOGEN. A substance or irritant that contribute to the development of cancer.
CARCINOMA. Any cancer that originates in the tissue that forms the skin or mucus membranes.
CAROTID. A major artery leading to the brain.
CATALYZE. A chemical reation of a substance that in itself remains unaffected.
CATHETER. Tube for passage through body channels usually to evacuate fluids.
CHELATION. A chemical binding reaction by pulling out or withdrawing.
COLESTEROL. Substance, a steroid found in fats and oils.
CLAUDICATION. A pain in the calf of the leg, from artery acclusion.
COAGULATION. Formation of a blood clot.
COENZYME. Non protein substance which activates an enzyme.
COLLAGEN. Fibers making up structural proteins in the body.
CROSS LINKAGE. One cell is chemically united to a neighboring cell by a bridge or bond between their atoms. A biological side reaction of a cell.
CYSTITIS. Inflammation of the bladder.
DIEURETIC. Medicine which increases the flow of urine.
DIVETICULITES. Inflammation of small pouches in the large intestine.
EFFICACY. Power to produce effects.
ENDARTERECTOMY. Incision of an artery, removal of material as in chelation therapy.
ENZYME. A protein with catalystic ability formed in living cells.
FATTY STREAK. A flat slightly elevated fat build up that does not narrow the vessels.
FIBROUS PLAQUE. A thick connective tissue containing various amounts of fats.
FREE RADICALS. Reactive molecular fragments generally harmful to the body, makes chain reactions.
GANGRENE. Death of tissue due to lack of blood.
GLYCEMIA. Sugar in the blood.
HYPEREMIA. Congestion of blood in a body organ resulting fro dialation or blockage.
IONIZATION. To give an electrical charge, put together or take apart by electrolysis.
ISCHEMIC. Insufficient circulation, local anemia, lack of blood.
LIPID. Fat like substance.
METABOLISM. The building up and breaking down processes of the body as a whole.
MYOCARDIAL INFRACTION. Blood clot or injury of middle layer of the heart wall. Dead tissue.
NECLEIC ACIDS. A chemical substance in cells such as DNA RNA
OCCLUSION. The closing of a passage.
PERICARDIUM. Sac inclosing the heart.
PEROXIDATION. Tissue aging, more oxide than any other.
PLATELETS. Disc shaped structure found in the blood for coagulation.
PLERITIS. Ulceration, pigmentation or dermatitis in thrombosis of the veins.
PLETHYSMOGRAPHY. Technique measures blood flow externally.
POLYSACHARIDE. A complete carbohydrate.
RENAL. Pertaining to the kidneys.
RETINOPATHY. Any non inflammatory disease of the retina.
SCLEROSIS. Hardening of tissue or organ.
SCHIZOPHERENIA. Emotional disorder, retreat from reality, delusions, hallucinations.
TRUAMA. Physical bruse, fracture or sprain. injury to subconcious due to emotional shock.
UREMIA. A toxic condition of the blood due to paisoning from urinary substances in blood.
VARICOSE VEINS. Swollen veins caused by improper valve function.
VASODEPRESSOR. Agent which relaxes the blood pressure.
VASOMOTOR. Influencing the contraction and dialation of blood vessels.
VITAMIN. Chemical substance found in foods that are necessary for proper body function.

ADDITIONAL READER HELP AND ORDERING FORM

FULL TEXT OF REPORTED SCIENTIFIC INFORMATION REPORTED IN CHAPTERS.

CHELATION THERAPY'S CORRECTION TO BIOLOGICAL AGING.
Full text of presentation to Prolongation of life.
By Donald G. Carpenter, Ph.D. $3.35

HOW TO ATTAIN TOTAL WELLNESS
A patients guide to Holistic Preventive medicine and including questions and answers on Chelation therapy.
By Robert A. Gegan 1.75

HAIR ANALYSIS, ITS CURRENT USES AND LIMITATIONS
By Garry F. Gordon, M.D. 3.00

HISTORY AND MECHANISM OF ACTION OF EDTA AND CHELATION THERAPY.
By Garry F. Gordon M.D. 3.00

EDTA CHELATION THERAPY II, EFFICACY IN BRAIN DISORDERS.
By H. Richard Casdorph M.D. Ph.D. 4.00
PRESENTED IN FALL EDITION OF *JOURNAL OF HOLISTIC MEDICINE 1981*

THE STORY OF CHELATION THERAPY.
By W. W. Holderby M.D. 2.00

Make check or money order payable to
CIP BOOKS
P.O. BOC 6203
Clearwater, Fl 33518

Include 65 cents postage for each booklet for postage and handling. May also be charged to Visa or Master charge.

VISA ☐ MASTERCHARGE ☐

Credit Card Orders Only

Total charges $ ________ Fill in the boxes below.

Credit Card No.

Expiration Date Month/Year

Name—First, Last

Street address

Company name or additional address line

City

State

ZIP Code

(or County)

READER'S INVITATION FOR SUPPORT FOR CONGRESSIONAL OR CONSTITUTIONAL REFORM FOR FREEDOM OF MEDICAL CHOICE

TO: The Executive and legislative branches of the Government.

With our mounting concern for our health maintenance costs and government policies toward organized medicine, WE THE UNDERSIGNED petition that legislative and constitutional reform take place to reverse our financial and health care predicament.

WHERAS: Our concern is the staggering and rising costs of medical care, we seek to promote a program to CUT the cost of illness and disease. We know that most major illness and disease are predictable and preventable before the major cost of such health care takes over. We need these savings eneacted into a program now.

WHERAS: The congress in 1962 hastily passed the Kefauver-Harris Amendment. In doing so the too-strict guidelines of the FDA now control the health of the American people to the point of financial bankrupcy. We suggest concentrating on the following points in your legislative activity.

1. The elimination of the need for efficacy and control studies and the substitution of such ideas as statistical proof or limit the FDA guidelines to safety alone.

2. Allow the use of Chelation Therapy and EDTA in the less expensive control of coronary artery disease and the use of the therapy in prevention of coronary disease and many other allied diseases.

3. Support the MEDICAL FREEDOMS BILL HR 983 by Dr. Lawrence P. McDonald Atlanta. Therby giving freedom of medical choice to all Americans as well as altering the FDA guidelines to control safety alone.

4. Seek the advice of the representatives of ALL the medical professions and prominant scientists in a national conference on PREVENTION OF ILLNESS and the promotion of a NATIONAL HEALTH REFORMATION. Resolve that the AMA has no monopoly on government, laws, or medical wisdom.

WHERAS: The American people are rising up in unified numbers to release the control of our lives and our health. We know this action poses bold action on your part, but we no longer will stand still to a medical lobby that is slowly destroying our will and our pocketbook. We assure you that this united action will be fought at the ballot box as well. We look forward to seeing your mind and spirit rise in unison as ours in now doing.

SIGNED ______________________ PRINT NAME ______________________
PRINT ADDRESS ____
COUNTY ____________________ STATE ____________________ ZIP ________

SIGNED ______________________ PRINT NAME ______________________
PRINT ADDRESS ____
COUNTY ____________________ STATE ____________________ ZIP ________

IMPORTANT NOTE:

We need your help and support two ways........

1. To add your names and addresses to our long list of petitioners.
   Direct a postcard to AFFOMC P.O. Box 6203 Clearwater, Fl. 33518
   Saying "Please add these names to your Alliance For Freedom Of Medical Choice petition" Sign and then print again your name and address legibly as it appears on the petition (above)

2. Also write your own letters to your Senators and representative in your State and district. Use your own words from the above text. This is always an effective means of political communication.

You will be glad you took this time to help secure your health standards.